CIRCUMCISION EXPOSED

Rethinking a Medical and Cultural Tradition

by Billy Ray Boyd

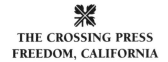

THE CROSSING PRESS
FREEDOM, CALIFORNIA

For information on bulk purchases or group discounts for this and other
Crossing Press titles, please contact our Special Sales Manager at 800-777-1048.

Visit our Website on the Internet at: www.crossingpress.com

Cataloging-in-Publication Data

Boyd, Billy Ray.
   [Circumcision, what it does]
   Exposing circumcision : rethinking a medical and cultural tradition / By Billy
Ray Boyd.
      p cm.
     Originally published : Circumcision. San Francisco : Taterhill Press, 1990.
     Includes bibliographical references (p.).
     ISBN 0-89594-939-3 (pbk.)
     1. Circumcision. 2. Circumcision—Social aspects. 3. Circumcision—
Psychological aspects. 4. Infants—Surgery.
     I. Title.
     RD590.B69 1998
     617.4'63--dc21   97-52376
                                                  CIP

I lovingly dedicate this book to the courageous wounded warriors who, with little support and in the face of trivialization, misinformation, and widespread denial, carry on the fight to end the sexual mutilation of children.

ACKNOWLEDGMENTS

I thank Marilyn Milos for my initiation into this painful and liberating knowledge; Tim Hammond for his understanding of social change and for keeping me up to date; Jill Schettler, Kendra Morrison, and Sweeney Schragg at The Crossing Press for believing in this book; Clay Olson for his dedicated support in getting this book into print; and Paulann Sternberg, Frederick Hodges, Tina Kimmel, Arla Ertz, Ed Duvin, Rosemary Romberg, Charan van Tijn, John Erickson, Marti Kheel, and others too numerous to mention, for their various contributions.

To those in co-counseling circles and the nonviolent direct action movements for peace, justice, and planetary survival I am grateful for their insights into gender issues, religious circumcision, and anti-Semitism.

CONTENTS

FOREWORD

Babies are a miracle. They come complete and perfect with all their functional parts ready to develop into a total human being. It is our job as parents, teachers, and others to guide them in their growth and development to become the best they can be—to become intelligent, compassionate, healthy individuals in mind, body, and spirit.

A baby is born into an imperfect world, yet he or she is pure and full of trust. A baby's wants and needs are simple. A baby needs nourishment—not only physical, but emotional nourishment. S/he wants to be held and hugged and loved and kissed and touched, to hear music—soothing and gentle sounds—like those produced by a harp, cello, or human voice.

It seems absurd that today we choose to mutilate a significant percentage of our newborn infants. As a young medical student in the 1960s, I learned the technique of performing the surgical procedure of male circumcision. It was not difficult to learn this procedure, and I very rapidly became expert at removing the foreskin from a newborn. I was able to do circumcisions in a very short amount of time—four or five minutes. I did this at the parents' request, and I was oblivious to the infant's cry.

Several years later into my pediatrics career, after having performed perhaps a hundred circumcisions, I became aware of the newborn's pain that I had somehow managed to put out of my consciousness. I now know that every baby that I circumcised cried and that I never responded to their pain. I then decided I was on their side; my job was to protect babies, not harm them. It was only then that I began my study of the foreskin, how it is unlike any tissue found elsewhere in the human body and accordingly, has special functions. The doctors and others performing this procedure on newborn babies do not know the pain they are causing nor do they appreciate the functions of that unique bit of tissue.

Billy Ray Boyd, in writing this book, will have a profound impact on a ritual more than 2,000 years old that has been based on superstition, tradition, and religious beliefs, with little basis in medicine. This book will change outmoded methods of thinking. Parents, doctors, and religious leaders will learn from this book and come away from it with regret that this procedure was done to them and done by them.

It is understandable that parents, doctors, and religious leaders have always wanted what is best for their children. It is only by changing this practice that we will stop hurting our babies in a manner that cannot be good for them. Circumcision not only destroys an important part of anatomy and, therefore, the male's physiology, but also psychologically and emotionally damages him.

Infants do feel pain. This has been proven without a doubt in many recent studies. To continue to perform this procedure on our babies without medical justification is a practice that should and will end. This book will make that end come sooner rather than later.

Paul M. Fleiss, M.D.

Paul Fleiss, M.D., *has been a practicing pediatrician in Hollywood for over thirty years. He has treated over 30,000 patients, including the children of some of Hollywood's most famous stars. Dr. Fleiss is an Assistant Clinical Professor of Pediatrics at USC School of Medicine, a Clinical Professor of Pediatrics at College of Osteopathic Medicine of the Pacific, and a lecturer at UCLA School of Public Health. He is on the medical advisory board for La Leche League International and also on the advisory board for the National Organization of Circumcision Information Resource Centers.*

INTRODUCTION

We love our children. Though we often make mistakes, we strive to give them the best support possible. We want them to be healthy and loving. We want them to be independent and also carry on that which is good and useful in our family and cultural traditions. Most of us do not want to harm our children. Parents who have their babies circumcised generally have the well-being of the children in mind.

My exploration of this subject began unexpectedly a few years ago. I was reading an article on circumcision practices around the world when I became so nauseated I couldn't continue reading. I didn't know why I felt that way, and at the time I didn't care to find out—my feelings were too intense.

A year or two later, I discovered the National Organization of Circumcision Information Resource Centers (NOCIRC). I read their material and established a correspondence and later a friendship with its founder and director, a registered nurse with three circumcised sons and an uncircumcised grandson. I became aware of my own submerged feelings about my circumcision and learned the medical and cultural history of the practice.

In the following pages, I discuss circumcision in terms of history, health, religion, economics, politics, parental and infant rights, and sexuality. I address the topics of ritual circumcision. I explore circumcision not only in medical, historical, and anthropological terms, but also from a personal perspective as a circumcised man.

For further information, see the Resources listed at the end of this book. I have relied especially on Rosemary Romberg's *Circumcision: The Painful Dilemma*, which I refer to in these pages simply as "Romberg." Unfortunately, it is out of print, as is Bruno Bettelheim's *Symbolic Wounds: Puberty Rites and the Envious Male*, which I also refer to. Readers can usually obtain copies of these books through inter-library loan programs of local libraries, and Romberg's book may be coming out on CD-ROM. Perhaps the best affordable resource on the subject is the video "Whose Body, Whose Rights?" which intelligently depicts all aspects of both medical and ritual circumcision.

I think it's important that I explain my use of terms and—when my usage is not standard—why I choose them. "Circumcisionist" means a person who advocates the routine practice of circumcision, especially on minors. "Circumciser" means one who actually performs circumcisions. I have used, instead of "anti-circumcision(ist)," the term "sexual preservationist," or "preservationist," to refer to a person, organization, policy, etc., opposed to involuntary circumcision. I have used the term "intact" in place of "uncircumcised." To refer to the movement against involuntary circumcision, I use the term "preservationist movement."

To circumcise (from the Latin, "to cut around") means to cut off part or all of the foreskin of a penis, permanently exposing the normally covered glans—or, with females, to surgically remove the clitoral hood.

In giving talks and facilitating workshops, I've discovered that some people—especially those who support infant circumcision—initially react defensively to terms like "genital mutilation" when applied to practices of their own culture.

"Genital Mutilation," a term commonly used in anthropology, refers to any whole or partial removal of human genitalia. It's also more accurate than "circumcision" in describing the broad range of what is done to male and female genitalia in various cultures.

The term "genital cutting" covers the whole range of female and male circumcision also, but avoids using the emotionally loaded negative term "mutilation." It applies to both males and females and provides an alternative to the term "circumcision," which has become too clinical a term.

I tend to use the term "sexual mutilation" most frequently, following the lead of the organizers of the 1996 Fourth International Symposium on Sexual Mutilations, in previous years called the International Symposia on Circumcision. Such direct terminology is scientifically accurate, honors the feelings of the victims of the practice, does an end-run around cultural denial and rationalization, and speaks to the sexual price inherent in this practice. I use the term because it emphasizes an essential focus for the preservationist movement—the impact that infant circumcision has on adult sexuality, both for the one circumcised and for his sexual partners. I use the term "circumcision" sometimes in its narrow sense of foreskin removal, and sometimes in the broader sense to mean any alteration of genitalia. I have tried to make sure that in each case the context makes clear which meaning is intended.

I use masculine pronouns only when referring specifically to males. When I refer to a person whose gender is unknown or is not specific, I use "they," "them," and "their." Such use has a long history among all social classes as well as widespread current usage.

I often use the adjective "ritual" for what is usually called "religious" circumcision. I do so to emphasize that Jewish, Moslem, and other religious circumcision practices are cultural phenomena. In doing so, I am not implying that ritual is necessarily uncivilized. Our lives can be greatly enriched by rituals. I also avoid the term "religious," because it is often used to seal off a belief or practice from critical scrutiny, whereas the purpose of this book is to examine all aspects of circumcision.

The term "fundamentalist" can have two very different meanings. It can mean finding and living by the essential fundamentals of a belief system (like truth, love, compassion), or it can refer to an acceptance of some (usually written) religious authority as infallible, not subject to interpretation in the light of changing social and historical conditions. I use the term in the latter sense. Christian and Islamic fundamentalism and Jewish orthodoxy share much in common, along with political fundamentalists of the right and left who follow their party lines without question.

I use the term "spiritual" and "spirituality" to refer to personal experience of and inquiry into the nature of self and life, and "religious" and "religion" to refer to a set of more-or-less fixed beliefs, dogmas, and/or rituals.

I sometimes use the term "involuntary circumcision" instead of the more usual "infant" or "routine circumcision" to emphasize the lack of consent on the part of the patient.

I've restricted discussion of religious circumcision mostly to Judaism. Jewish circumcision provided the model for medical circumcision as we know it. Some of the points I make refer equally to Islamic (or other socio-religious) circumcision, others not. For more information on male and female circumcision in Islamic cultures, see the Resources section at the end of this book.

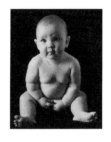

CIRCUMCISION, AN OVERVIEW

■ MALE CIRCUMCISION

Statistics

Did you know?

- Infant circumcision is the most commonly performed surgery in the U.S.—3,300 a day.

- At a cost of $500 to $800 million per year,[1] 58 percent of baby boys born in the U.S.—over a million every year—are currently being circumcised. This figure is lower than the figure of 90 percent in the 1960s. In the western states, a majority of baby boys are now being left intact. In the future, *circumcised* boys and men in the U.S. will be seen as different from the norm—as they are in Europe and most of the world today.

- Estimates of complications from circumcision vary widely, depending on the definition of the word "complication" and also on the accuracy of medical records on botched circumcisions. Between 2 and 10 percent is probably accurate.[2] Documented infection and complications have led to impotence, loss of the penis's shaft skin, convulsions, massive brain and kidney damage, quadriplegia, and death. Even the late circumcisionist Aaron J. Fink, M.D., acknowledged two to three U.S. deaths per year from circumcision. Other estimates range as high as 200 deaths per year in the U.S.

- Infants' penises have been lost in a slip of a knife—two in one day in 1985 in a Georgia hospital. One of these babies was subsequently converted into a girl and will need to take hormones for the rest of his/her life. Botched circumcisions have created, in the words of a past President of the Virginia Urologic Society, "lifetime genital cripples."

- Many men circumcised in adulthood report a lessening of the sensitivity of the penis, starting soon afterward or two or three years later. This desensitization is probably greater in infant circumcision, due to the ripping apart of the foreskin and glans (head of penis) prior to the surgery. In adults, they have already naturally separated.

- Foreskin restoration is possible either through surgery or by applying gentle skin expansion techniques to what is left of the foreskin. Both have been practiced for thousands of years.

The Reality of Infant Circumcision

> The maltreatment of children has existed since recorded time, and has taken many forms...Children were mutilated for a variety of reasons. Circumcision, foot and head binding, and castration were all accepted at various times in history.
>
> —Norman S. Ellerstein, M.D.
> *Child Abuse and Neglect: A Medical Reference*[3]

On any given day, in any U.S. city, baby boys are strapped down with velcro restraints on molded plastic boards, actually brand-named "Circumstraints," specifically designed to hold them immobile while their most sensitive tissues are efficiently and traumatically sliced off. The surgery usually happens in the nursery, or a room nearby.

After the baby is strapped down, an antiseptic is applied to the genital area, and a paper or cloth drape is placed over the baby's body with a hole exposing the genitals, much like a rubber dental dam is used by a dentist to obscure all parts of the mouth except the tooth being worked on. Before it can be cut off, the baby's foreskin has to be separated from the glans. (If left alone, they separate gently and naturally over a number of years.) A probe is forced under the foreskin and moved around the glans, tearing them apart. This is when the baby usually starts to scream, unless he goes quickly into shock. The loosened foreskin is then slit with surgical scissors. The screams intensify, and the baby's heart rate increases dramatically. He may go into a comatose state to escape

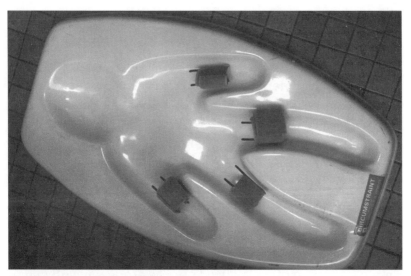

Circumstraint board.

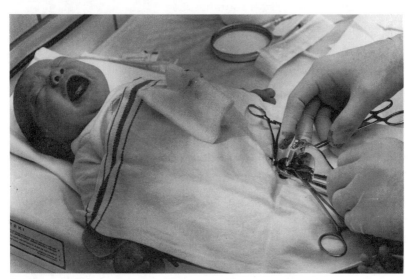

Infant responding to circumcision procedure.

the pain, a state often mistaken for sleep. Some babies vomit or defecate. What happens next depends on the type of device used. In one procedure, a little cone or "bell" device is then placed over the raw glans to protect it. The foreskin is stretched over the outside of the cone and tied, then cut off, circular fashion, around the cone, with a scalpel. Alternatively, the Gomco clamp can be used to crush the foreskin against the cone for three to five minutes, lessening bleeding while the foreskin is amputated. The wound is dressed and the baby begins a healing period of up to a week. His penis is swollen and tender, urine burns the wound, and the abrasion of diapers causes additional pain and discomfort. If a Plastibell device is used, it is left on for a week to ten days until the foreskin, deprived of a blood supply, dies and falls off.

So What's the Big Deal?

In a country like the U.S. where the great majority of men are circumcised, concern over the practice—and especially its implications for sexuality—is often viewed as making a mountain out of a molehill. "I'm doing fine with sex," a typical circumcised man will say. "So what's the big deal?"

The "big deal" has been understood for a very long time. Recognizing the sexual role of the foreskin, the great eleventh-century Jewish philosopher and physician Moses Maimonides succinctly stated that the effect—indeed, the primary purpose—of infant male circumcision was as follows:

...to limit sexual intercourse, and to weaken the organ of generation as far as possible, and thus cause man to be moderate...for there is no doubt that circumcision weakens the power of sexual excitement, and sometimes lessens the natural enjoyment; the organ necessarily becomes weak when...deprived of its covering from the beginning.

—*Guide for the Perplexed*, Part III, Chapter XLIX

The foreskin (also called the prepuce) is a natural protective covering for the head (or glans) of the penis. The average adult male foreskin consists of one and one-half inches of outer skin and one and one-half inches of inner mucosal lining and is five inches in circumference when the penis is erect. Containing over 240 feet of nerves and over 1,000 nerve endings, the foreskin is the most densely nerve-laden part of the penis and therefore its most erogenous part. Infant circumcision removes all these nerves in what would in adulthood become about fifteen square inches of erogenous tissue. That's almost a four-inch square, constituting more than a third of an adult's penile shaft skin. Half of that, the inside of the foreskin, is extremely sensitive tissue. It's all sliced away in circumcision.

People with experience both ways—those circumcised as adults, and those who have successfully undergone foreskin restoration*—tend to agree that a penis with its slidable

*While the nerves cut away are gone forever, there are both surgical and non-surgical methods of restoring the foreskin, re-covering the glans so that it remoistens and resensitizes.

Inner and Outer Foreskin Layers

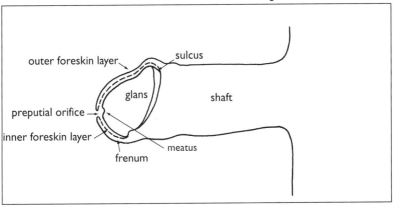

Circumcised Penis in Relaxed State

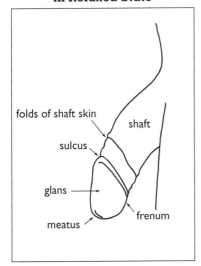

Uncircumcised Penis in Relaxed State

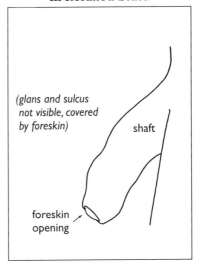

foreskin is more fun to play with and to *be* played with than a circumcised one. This contributes toward pleasure in masturbation and sexual play with a partner.

The foreskin keeps a man's penis naturally lubricated so that the glans stays moist and sensitive. And when the penis becomes erect, it pushes out of this nerve-laden sleeve of skin, so that what in the flaccid state is the sensitive inside of the foreskin becomes the outside skin of the lengthened penis, covering up to a third or more of the entire penis shaft. It is this tissue, with its capacity for pleasure when in contact with a partner's similar tissues, that circumcision slices away forever.

Paul M. Fleiss, M.D. identifies six known functions of the foreskin, while adding that there may well be additional functions not yet known: protection of the glans, immunological defense, erogenous sensitivity, coverage during erection, self-stimulating sexual functions, sexual functions in intercourse.

> The foreskin fosters intimacy between the two partners by enveloping the glans and maintaining it as an internal organ. The sexual experience is enhanced when the foreskin slips back to allow the male's internal organ, the glans, to meet the female's internal organ, the cervix—a moment of supreme intimacy and beauty."[4]

How much sexual sensitivity remains after circumcision also depends on how much of the *frenulum* (also called *frenum*) was cut away or left. This is the fold of mucous membrane that attaches to the glans and the inside of the foreskin on the underside of the penis to keep the foreskin over the

Erection Process of Circumcised Penis

Erection Process of Uncircumcised Penis

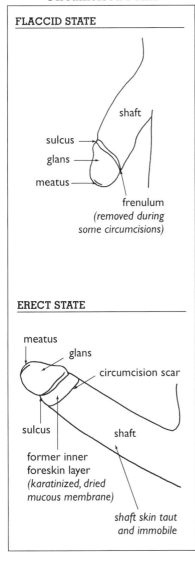

FLACCID STATE

shaft

sulcus

glans

meatus

frenulum
*(removed during
some circumcisions)*

ERECT STATE

meatus

glans

circumcision scar

sulcus

shaft

former inner
foreskin layer
*(karatinized, dried
mucous membrane)*

*shaft skin taut
and immobile*

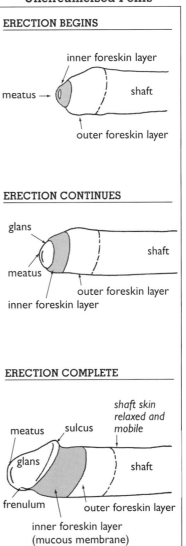

ERECTION BEGINS

inner foreskin layer

meatus →

shaft

outer foreskin layer

ERECTION CONTINUES

glans

shaft

meatus

outer foreskin layer

inner foreskin layer

ERECTION COMPLETE

*shaft skin
relaxed and
mobile*

meatus   sulcus

glans

shaft

frenulum

outer foreskin layer

inner foreskin layer
(mucous membrane)

glans except when pulled back. It's loaded with nerves. As one man described it, "I am not cut. All of my friends were, so I was very different. Even when I was very little and learned about circumcision, I wondered why something should be cut off that felt so good. After puberty I could make myself come by just rubbing my frenum between my thumb and index finger, so the sensitivity is unquestionable."[5] Varying degrees of the frenulum are cut away in circumcision. Many babies under the knife lose it all, some a chunk or two of their glans as well. A few babies lose their penises, their health, even their lives.

During over a hundred years of performing circumcisions, the medical profession never studied the consequences of the procedure. In 1996, an article by three Canadian doctors in the *British Journal of Urology* broke new ground. Titled "The Prepuce: Specialized Mucosa of the Penis and Its Loss to Circumcision," it concluded that, "The amount of tissue loss estimated in the present study is more than most parents envisage from pre-operative counseling. Circumcision also ablates junctional mucosa that appears to be an important component of the overall sensory mechanism of the human penis."[6] To put it in lay terms, parents don't have a clue how much skin will be sliced away when they sign the consent form, and sex is not as enjoyable without the tip of the foreskin, where the outside skin and the inside mucosal lining meet.

While it may be impossible for circumcised men to know what they are missing—and what the value of a foreskin would be—they may be able to get an idea. You'll probably notice that the circumcision scar is much more sensitive than even the glans itself. That's some indication of what the whole inside of the foreskin—which becomes, during erection, about a third of the outer shaft skin—might feel like if it hadn't been cut away.

But not all men respond this way; the scar can be either sensitive or numb. Romberg raises an interesting point: "Women complain that men are too "blunt" in their approach, "cut off" from their feelings...I suspect a connection [with circumcision]."[7] When we consider how obsessed with sex our society seems to be we have to wonder why our media, including feminist writers, have not explored this connection between circumcision, sexuality, and male desensitization.

Dr. Dean Edell, who gives medical advice on radio and television, is of the opinion that "future historians will find it incredible that in our day we mutilated babies by cutting off the end of their penises in the name of medicine. There are now serious concerns this may actually deprive men of a vital part of their sexuality." Dr. Edell is understating the issue. A decrease in sexuality was the explicit reason for the medical institution of circumcision in the first place.

Just as the foreskin protected the glans of early man from rough and thorny underbrush, today it protects men from the irritation of abrasive clothing and zippers. The permanently exposed glans of a circumcised penis dries up and develops, in the body's wisdom, a layer of nerveless skin called a *corneum*, which tries to perform the protective function of the foreskin. According to Dr. Dean Edell, the corneum is twelve to fifteen cell layers thick, compared with one or two layers for a glans constantly protected by a moist foreskin. This corneum separates the nerves in a man's glans from the moist, sensitive tissues of a sexual partner.

> The glans at birth is delicate and easily irritated by urine and feces. The foreskin shields the glans; with circumcision, this protection is lost. In such cases, the glans and especially the urinary opening (meatus) may become irritated or infected, causing ulcers, meatitis (inflammation of the meatus), and meatal stenosis (a narrowing of the urinary opening). Such problems virtually never occur in uncircumcised penises. The foreskin protects the glans throughout life.
>
> —American Academy of Pediatrics
> *Care of the Uncircumcised Penis* (brochure, 1984 version)

Visualizing the Operation

It's often difficult for a circumcised man—or a woman who has no experience with an uncircumcised partner—to visualize what a foreskin really is, and therefore to understand what its sexual function is. Here's how I make this clear when I speak on the subject.

Get a long-sleeved shirt with a snugly buttoning cuff. Slip an arm into one of the shirt sleeves, and button the cuff around your wrist. Hold this sleeved arm out in front of you, elbow bent at a right angle. Make a loose fist with the hand of this sleeved arm. With your other hand, tug the sleeve until your fist is covered with a double layer of shirt sleeve. Your forearm represents the shaft of a penis; the fist, the glans or head; and the shirt sleeve, the shaft skin and foreskin, which are continuous.

Place the thumb and index finger of your free hand around the wrist of the demonstration arm. Mark the line on the shirtsleeve where your fingers circle your wrist with chalk or a non-staining marker. Also mark or note the line where the sleeve folds and tucks back to become the inside of the fore-skin next to the glans.

When a penis becomes erect, it pushes out of its foreskin sleeve. You can simulate this by pulling back on the sleeve, until it's in the normal position of a shirt sleeve on an arm. Note that about two-thirds of the shaft skin of this erect penis was a moment ago foreskin on the flaccid penis. Half of that—about one-third of what is now shaft skin—is the *inside* of the foreskin in the flaccid state. On a human body, that skin is moist, highly sensitive mucous tissue, much like the inside of your eyelid or mouth. That tissue constitutes the most sensi-tive tissue on the shaft of the penis. When a man engages in intercourse, that tissue comes in contact with the moist, sen-sitive mucous tissues of his partner.

Now re-cover your fist with the shirtsleeve and imagine the circumcision procedure. In infants, the foreskin is attached to the glans (which isn't the case with the sleeve and your fist). The two must be ripped apart, arguably the most traumatic part of the whole procedure for a baby. You can simulate this by inserting a pencil between the glans and the foreskin, running it around the fist until the two are "separated," imagining the tearing apart of very sensitive tissues.

Next, the foreskin must be cut off. You don't need to do this to your shirt, of course, but use your imagination. Now, instead of having a lot of skin that will slide back and forth on the penis, you have a much tighter shaft skin. This is why it's said that circumcision removes the penis's only moving part, and takes a lot of the play out of foreplay.

FEMALE CIRCUMCISION

Statistics

A 1996 report out of Egypt revealed the following[8]:

- Women who are circumcised are more likely to have their daughters circumcised than women who are not circumcised.

- Women cite custom as the main factor in their decision to have their daughters circumcised. Husbands play no role, or only a marginal one, in the women's decisions.

- Women are shifting from traditional circumcisers to medical doctors to have their daughters circumcised.

- 16 percent of Egyptian women are circumcised by removing "only" the labia majora or minora, externalizing the clitoris much the same way that the male glans is externalized in male circumcision as we know it.

- 68 percent don't believe that it causes complications leading to death.

- 79 percent don't believe that it causes problems for conception or pregnancy.

- 79 percent don't believe that it can cause difficult labor.

- 47 percent don't believe that it decreases sexual satisfaction.

- 82 percent of married and previously married women fifteen to forty-nine years old believe that the practice should be continued.

Common Origins of Female and Male Circumcision

> Most people in Western society...find [female circumcision] repugnant. Yet the origins of female circumcision and the justifications for its practice are very much similar to those of male circumcision.
>
> —Rosemary Romberg,
> *Circumcision: The Painful Dilemma*

There are various theories about how male or female circumcision began in prehistoric cultures. In some cases it may have begun as a way to squelch divisiveness in a tribe or to enforce a sovereign's power over his subjects by forcing them to yield up their children. To go back further in time, it may have evolved from the practice of child sacrifice. Freudian psychologists theorized that when older dominant males mated with multiple younger females, the threat of genital mutilation kept younger men in line, resulting in the "castration complex" among the males. This theory is not currently in favor. Some claim that circumcision was perceived as a medical necessity for desert nomads with little water for men to wash themselves. It may have been a way of branding slaves. Some have argued that it was influenced by women wishing that men would bleed like them. It may have developed along with the domestication of animals and its psychology of domination and practice of biological manipulation (including castration).

My favorite theory is one propounded by Bruno Bettelheim in *Symbolic Wounds: Puberty Rites and the Envious Male*: Genital mutilations began as a rite of passage, a puberty rite, a product of male envy of girls' initiation into adulthood through menstruation and changed from an adolescent to an infant procedure with the development of monotheism. In almost all cultures that practice circumcision today, it is still a rite of passage performed on adolescents. It apparently occurs only in societies that are male-dominated. In every society that sexually mutilates females, male sexual mutilation apparently came first, though only a minority of cultures that do it to males also do it to females.

Female circumcision is usually, though not always, a more severe form of genital mutilation than male circumcision as practiced in the U.S. Some women working against these procedures in their own countries have reacted negatively to the use of the emotionally loaded term "genital mutilation" by horrified Westerners, maintaining that "circumcision" is a more acceptable word. A narrow definition of female circumcision would be the surgical removal of the clitoral hood, but the term is commonly used in a broader sense to include all female genital mutilations. This can be the cutting but nonremoval of the clitoral hood or the clitoris itself, *clitoridectomy* (removal of part or all of the clitoris), or, as is common in the Sudan, *vulvectomy* (removal of the inner and/or outer vaginal lips) with or without *infibulation* (sewing up of the vagina, leaving only a small opening for the passage of menstrual blood). A whole class of midwives and other women make their living performing these procedures. In Egypt, many untrained men perform clitoridectomies and male circumcisions in their street stalls. Despite this, many women assert their *right* to continue this practice on their daughters, because they live in societies where mutilation, with its enforcement of sexual docility, is a prerequisite for marriage and therefore for economic survival.

While female circumcision is not common in the West, removal of the clitoral hood has been prescribed by some doctors as a way to bring "unruly" sexual appetites under control and by others for the opposite effect, to increase sexual sensation by keeping the clitoris constantly exposed. Desmond Morris, in his book *Body Watching*, cites a Texas doctor who, as late as 1937, advocated removal of the clitoris as a cure for frigidity. The Winter 1989–90 issue of the *NOCIRC Newsletter*, in an item headed "Female Circumcision in America," cites other cases of female circumcision in the U.S.:

> In 1955, the clitoris and labia were removed from a 12-year old Baltimore girl who now, at 47, has just learned that the statute of limitations prevents her from taking legal action against the doctor who caused her physical and psychological damage.

> A gynecologist who performed experimental genital surgery on thirty-three women without their knowledge lost his license to practice last year after a CBS News report exposed his "love surgery." The experimental operations, including circumcision, resulted in complaints by the women of sexual dysfunction similar to complaints made by many circumcised men.

Worldwide, an estimated 2,000,000 girls per year are sexually mutilated, about 13,300,000 boys.[9] As with female genital mutilation, there is a wide range in what is or has been done to male children. This includes partial castration (removal of one testicle), infibulation of the foreskin over the glans to promote chastity, and *subincision* (slitting the entire underside of the penis to the urethra and splaying it out). Perhaps the most severe form of male circumcision, among the Yesidis in Vilajat Assir in Yemen, has been the "stripping of the skin from the navel to the anus, including the skin of the penis and scrotum of a young bridegroom."[10]

> The one being circumcised may not cry out nor wail or he would be despised and forsaken by his bride, who witnesses the procedure. Hot oil is put on the wound. People often die of the consequences, many leave the tribe.[11]

Comparison of Male and Female Circumcision

Before

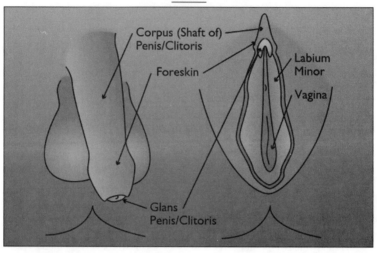

Corpus (Shaft of)
Penis/Clitoris

Foreskin

Labium
Minor

Vagina

Glans
Penis/Clitoris

After

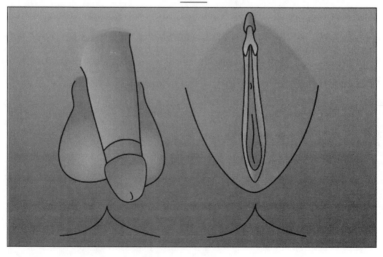

Only *male* mutilation has achieved the status of religious scriptural injunction, though there are certainly myths in various cultures which describe the sacred origins of female as well as male circumcision. In almost all cultures which circumcise males and/or females, it is performed on teens or pre-teens, as in Islam today. Male circumcision is nearly universal in Islamic cultures, whereas female circumcision is practiced in some but not others. Within one country, there can be heated debate about whether female circumcision is a proper expression of Islamic propriety. In Egypt in 1997 the head of the eminent Islamic institute, al-Azhar, issued a religious edict urging the government to execute anyone opposed to female circumcision. Human rights groups in turn sued the institute[12] and won a victory in the Egyptian Supreme Court. Dr. Nawal El Saadawi, the Egyptian physician who had been so active in the fight, then opened a new campaign against male circumcision.[13]

Wherever it's practiced, female circumcision tends to be more common among the poor, yet even a good number of the affluent, educated people continue the practice. In her book *Gyn Ecology: The Metaphysics of Radical Feminism*, Mary Daly writes of an interview with a young Egyptian woman physician who was expecting a baby.

> She said that if the child she was expecting should be a girl she would circumcise her herself. The young woman gave several reasons. The first was religious: she was a muslim [sic]. The second was cosmetic: she

wanted "to remove something disfiguring, ugly and repulsive." Thirdly, the girl should be protected from sexual stimulation through the clitoris. The fourth reason was tradition.[14]

Unlike most Westerners who have their sons circumcised, this woman was prepared to perform the operation on her daughter personally "for her own good." (As a physician, she was presumably medically qualified.) For this degree of forthrightness about *male* circumcision we have to turn to the anti-masturbation crusades of a hundred years ago, because in the West today it is not done with the intent (at least not the conscious intent) to decrease sexuality.

Female genital mutilation abroad and in some immigrant cultures has long been a feminist concern in the West, while less attention has been paid to male genital mutilation. Britain banned female circumcision with an Act of Parliament, while France applied already-existing child abuse laws to accomplish the same goal. In Italy, the national health service stirred up a storm of controversy by deciding to perform clitoridectomies on request, on the grounds that if they didn't, parents would have the procedure done at home with all the attendant risks.[15] Though many immigrants who practiced female circumcision stop when they come to the U.S., not all do. (The ones who practiced male circumcision usually continue.) As this book goes to press, state after state is passing laws against female sexual mutilation. In 1996 it became illegal under U.S. law to circumcise, excise, or infibulate all or any part of the labia majora or minora or clitoris of any person under eighteen years of age. (The law actually reads *person*, not *female*.)

Calling for an End to All Genital Mutilation

In the U.S., circumcision is clearly a men's issue, but it also has implications for women. It is the most basic maternal instinct to want to protect one's baby from physical harm. Routine circumcision overrides this instinct. It alters the physical sensations of sex for women as well as men. Most Americans, men and women, are as unaware of the negative consequences of male circumcision as people in many Arabic and African countries are unaware of the negative consequences of female circumcision.

In recent years, the U.S. public and medical professions have been shaken out of their complacency and gained a new perspective on male circumcision, because increasing immigration from Central African, Islamic, and Arabic countries has brought the topic of female circumcision into political debate. The public outcry creates a unique opportunity for the preservationist movement to help open people's eyes and hearts to the tragedy of *all* genital mutilation, male as well as female, at home as well as abroad. A number of leading activists have spoken and written about the connections between female and male sexual mutilation, including Alice Walker; Somalian filmmaker Soraya Mire (*Fire Eyes*); Egyptian physician Nawal El Saadawi; Shamis Dirir, Coordinator of the London Black Women's Health Action Project; and Sudanese physician Nahid Toubia. Born in Egypt, Dr. Toubia became the first woman surgeon in Sudan. She has been active in both medical and human rights struggles, including the fight to end female sexual mutilation. When a radio interviewer attempted to dissociate female genital mutilation from male circumcision, she disagreed:

> Interviewer: [I]n the communities where female genital mutilation occurs, it is often referred to as female circumcision. However, this term implies an analogy with male circumcision, which is not the case. Could you explain the difference?

> Toubia: Well, I disagree with you that it's not the case. I think there are similarities and then there are differences. I think the people who say that there are no similarities are people who don't want to address male circumcision.[16]

Dr. Toubia wrote in the *International Journal of Gynecology & Obstetrics:*

> The unnecessary removal of a functioning body organ in the name of tradition, custom, or any other non-disease related cause should never be acceptable to the health profession. All childhood circumcisions are violations of human rights and a breach of the fundamental code of medical ethics...

> It is the moral duty of educated professionals to protect the health and rights of those with little or no social power to protect themselves.[17]

BOYS & GIRLS—A CIRCUMCISION COMPARISON[18]

	Boys	Girls
Is the practice rooted in ancient blood ritual?	Yes	Yes
Was it initially adopted to suppress or control sexuality?	Yes	Yes
Did the practice become, or is it becoming, "medicalized"?	Yes	Yes
Do cultures use hygiene, medicine, religion, or tradition to justify it?	Yes	Yes
Is it done without anesthesia, and is it painful and traumatic to the child?	Yes	Yes
Does it carry long-term physical, sexual, emotional or psychological effects?	Yes	Yes
Does it diminish sexual sensitivity?	Yes	Yes
Does it abuse or mutilate the child's body?	Yes	Yes
Is it forced upon the child without his/her consent?	Yes	Yes
Do the victims learn to accept it as "normal" or defend the practice?	Yes	Yes
Do Americans widely condemn it?	No	Yes
Do Americans widely practice it?	Yes	No

WEAVING OUR VOICES

The following is an interweaving of two experiences. The roman text (non-italicized) is an account by Nawal El Saadawi, M.D., of her circumcision at age eight, from her book *The Hidden Face of Eve: Women in the Arab World*. Dr. Saadawi was fired as director of education in the Egyptian Ministry of Health and editor of *Health* magazine for publishing the book *Women and Sex*. The italicized text is from an account of the first circumcision witnessed by Marilyn Fayre Milos, during her training to become a midwife. The experience she describes launched her into her life's work to end the circumcision of baby boys.

I was six years old that night when I lay in my bed, warm and peaceful in the pleasurable state which lies halfway between wakefulness and sleep. I felt something like a huge hand, cold and rough, fumbling over my body, as though looking for something. Almost simultaneously another hand, as cold and as rough and as big as the first one, was clapped over my mouth, to prevent me from screaming.

We students filed into the newborn nursery to find a baby strapped spread-eagle to a plastic board on a counter top across the room. He was struggling against his restraints—tugging, whimpering, and then crying help-lessly.

They carried me to the bathroom. I do not know how many of them there were, nor do I remember their faces, or whether they were women or men.

No one was tending the infant, but when I asked my instructor if I could comfort him, she said, "Wait till the doctor gets here." I wondered how a teacher of the heal-ing arts could watch someone suffer and not offer assis-tance. I wondered about the doctor's power which could intimidate others from following protective instincts.

Something like an iron grasp caught hold of my hand, and my arms, and my thighs, so that I became unable to resist or even to move. I also remember the icy touch of the bathroom tiles under my naked body and unknown voices and humming sounds interrupted now and again by a rasping metallic sound which reminded me of the butcher when he used to sharpen his knife before slaugh-tering sheep.

When he did arrive, I immediately asked the doctor if I could help the baby. He told me to put my finger into the baby's mouth; I did, and the baby sucked. I stroked his lit-tle head and spoke softly to him. He began to relax, and was momentarily quiet.

I strained my ears trying to catch the metallic, rasping sound. The moment it ceased, I felt as though my heart had stopped beating, too. I was unable to see, and somehow my breathing seemed to have stopped. Yet I imagined the rasping sound coming closer and closer to me. Somehow it was not approaching my neck as I had expected, but another part of my body, somewhere below my belly, as though seeking something buried between my thighs. At that very moment, I realized that my thighs had been pulled wide apart, and that each of my legs was being held as far away from the other as possible, as though gripped by steel fingers that never relinquished their pressure. Then suddenly the sharp metallic edge dropped between my thighs...

The silence was broken by a piercing scream—the baby's reaction to having his foreskin pinched and crushed as the doctor attached the clamp to his penis.

...and cut off a piece of flesh from my body.

The shriek intensified when the doctor inserted an instrument between the foreskin and the head of the penis, tearing the two structures apart.

I screamed with pain despite the tight hand held over my mouth.

The baby started shaking his head back and forth—the only part of his body free to move—as the doctor used another clamp to crush the foreskin lengthwise, where he then cut. This made the opening of the foreskin large enough to insert a circumcision instrument.

The pain was like a searing flare that went through my whole body.

The baby began to gasp and choke, breathless from his shrill, continuous screams. My bottom lip began to quiver, tears filled my eyes and spilled over, I found my own sobs difficult to contain.

After a few moments, I saw a red pool of blood around my hips.

During the next stage of the surgery, the doctor crushed the foreskin against the circumcision instrument and then, finally, amputated it. The baby was limp, exhausted, spent.

I did not know what they had cut off, and I did not try to find out.

I had not been prepared, nothing could have prepared me, for this experience.

I just wept, and called out to my mother for help.

To see a part of this baby's penis being cut off was devastating.

But the worst shock of all was when I looked around and found her standing by my side.

But even more shocking was the doctor's comment, barely audible several octaves below the piercing screams of the baby: "There's no medical reason for doing this."

Yes, it was she. In flesh and blood, right in the midst of these strangers. She was talking to them, and smiling at them, as though they had not just participated in slaughtering her daughter.

I couldn't believe my ears, my knees became weak, and I felt sick to my stomach. I couldn't believe that medical professionals, dedicated to helping and healing, could inflict such unnecessary pain and anguish on innocent babies.

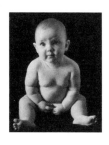

"MEDICAL" BASIS FOR CIRCUMCISION

AN OPERATION IN SEARCH OF A DISEASE

In all cases [of masturbation],...circumcision is undoubtedly the physicians' closest friend and ally... There must be no play in the skin after the wound has thoroughly healed, but it must fit tightly over the penis, for should there be any play the patient will be found to readily resume his practice, not begrudging the time and extra energy required to produce the orgasm. It is true, however, that the longer it takes to have an orgasm, the less frequently it will be attempted, consequently the greater the benefit gained.

—*Medical Record*, 1895[1]

Tying the hands is also successful in some cases... Covering the organs with a cage has been practiced with entire success. A remedy which is almost always successful in small boys is circumcision...The operation should be performed by a surgeon without administering an anesthetic, as the brief pain attending the operation will have a salutary effect upon the mind, especially if it be connected with the idea of punishment.

—John Kellogg,
health reformer and founder of Kellogg's Cereals™, 1888[2]

It wasn't until the last century that circumcision was advocated for a supposedly medical reason: to discourage masturbation. Some doctors thought masturbation caused or aggravated numerous medical problems including asthma, insanity, alcoholism, epilepsy, enuresis, hernia, gout, rectal prolapse, rheumatism, headaches, curvature of the spine, hip disease, hydrocephalus, and kidney disease. The theory was that sexual expression depleted one's limited lifetime allotment of vital energy; to use it for anything other than procreation was to invite degenerative diseases of all kinds.

Patients suffering the ravages of poverty, overwork, malnutrition, and various abuses attributed to the Industrial Revolution exhibited a range of pathologies. When doctors took patients' medical histories, and found that they had masturbated, the theory that masturbation caused the conditions was repeatedly "proven".

Circumcision *did* reduce the sensitivity of the penis and reduced the pleasure of masturbation, but eventually it became apparent that cutting off the penis's only moving part would not stop masturbation. As a result, doctors gradually stopped doing circumcisions *for this reason*. But instead of halting the practice, they came up with new reasons for it— cervical cancer, cancer of the penis, and so on—each reason replacing another as soon as it became discredited.

There has been no shortage of examples of knife-happy doctors past and present. We only need to look at the number of sometimes unnecessary surgeries like cesarean deliveries.

But while previous dubious medical practices—from blood-letting to routine tonsillectomy—have been dropped, circumcision has become more entrenched. Some say it's because this operation deals with the genitals, and that as members of a sexually repressive culture, we're less open to look carefully at the pros and cons of this operation. Others say that doctors may not want to admit they've been doing something wrong or lose the money they make from this quick operation. Some doctors sincerely believe what they're doing is right, others openly admit they're in it for the money. A surprising number don't want to circumcise babies, but are afraid that if they don't do it at the parents' request, they'll lose those whole families to other doctors who will.

In addition to the long-standing lucrativeness of the procedure itself, there are now financial benefits in *marketing* the foreskins of babies.[3]

> ...the marketing of purloined baby foreskins is a multi-million-dollar-a-year industry. Pharmaceutical companies use human foreskins as research material. Corporations such as Advanced Tissue Sciences, Organogenesis, and BioSurface Technology use human foreskins as the raw material for a type of breathable bandage.[4]

An example of the medical profession's approval of circumcision came in 1987 when the California Medical Association declared—in a resolution adopted *against the advice of its own board*—that circumcision is an "effective public health measure."

Only in English-speaking countries was widespread circumcision ever adopted for supposed medical reasons. However, in recent decades the medical professions in Britain, Australia, and New Zealand—everywhere except the U.S.— have moved away from the practice. According to the National Organization of Circumcision Information Resource Centers, the circumcision rates in those countries are now down to 1 percent, 18 percent, and 2 percent, respectively.

In the early editions of his book *Baby and Child Care*, Benjamin Spock, M.D., recommended infant circumcision. In later editions he changed his stand, and then, in the April, 1989, issue of *Redbook* magazine, in an article titled "Circumcision—It's Not Necessary," he stated, "My own preference, if I had the good fortune to have another son, would be to leave his little penis alone." Dr. Dean Edell also counsels viewers against circumcision.

Unfortunately, not all doctors have gotten the message. The result is that the U.S. is now the only country in the world in which non-religious circumcision is still widespread.

Though circumcision is essentially a cultural phenomenon, the reasons given for it today are largely medical. Because of this, it is necessary to deal briefly with the circumcisionists' main medical arguments before going on to the more relevant cultural and psychological aspects.

Cervical cancer. The idea that circumcision helps prevent cervical cancer arose around 1910 when it was noted that Jewish women had substantially lower incidences of cervical cancer than gentile women. Since circumcision in the non-Jewish population was not common at the time, and since almost all Jewish men were circumcised, it was assumed that somehow the presence of a foreskin—perhaps something it harbored—was linked to cervical cancer and, conversely, that circumcision prevented it.

Since 57 percent of U.S. males, Jews and non-Jews, are presently circumcised, we can now compare our cervical cancer rates with Europe's, where circumcision is rare. There is no significant difference, indicating that circumcision has no relevance to cancer of the cervix. So why are the incidences of cervical cancer lower in Jewish women? It may be the result of genetic factors. At any rate, few doctors these days take the idea seriously that cutting off a baby boy's foreskin will help prevent cervical cancer in a boy's future wife or sexual partners. Most would agree with the American Academy of Pediatrics that "Neonatal circumcision is unproven as a means of reducing...carcinoma of the cervix in marital partners..."[5]

Prostate cancer. In the U.S., prostate cancer has been a fairly common cause of death among men. In the 1940s, higher rates of prostate cancer were observed among gentiles than among Jews, giving rise to the theory that circumcision prevented prostate cancer.[6] When factors such as age, heredity, and environment were later taken into consideration, the theory no longer held. Whether the males in the study were circumcised evidently had no relevance to these cancer rates.

The American Academy of Pediatrics finally laid the question to rest in its typically understated manner:

> There is presently no convincing scientific evidence to substantiate the assertion that circumcision reduces the eventual incidence of cancer to the prostate.[7]

Urinary tract infections (UTI). According to a well-publicized study done in the late 1980s by Dr. T. E. Wiswell in U.S. military hospitals, UTIs occur at a rate of 1.4 in every hundred intact boys, compared with 0.14 in every hundred circumcised boys. In other words, intact boys, according to this study, are ten times more likely to get UTIs than are circumcised boys.

After Wiswell's results were published, a group of doctors from the pediatric departments of five different Swedish hospitals, writing in the British medical journal *The Lancet*,[8] suggested that any increase in the incidence of UTI among intact babies is due to the hospital birthing environment, not the foreskin. In a supposedly sterile hospital environment, the underforeskin area can very soon become colonized with harmful organisms such as hostile strains of *E Coli*, bacteria to which the baby has not developed an immunity. Once these bacteria set up permanent housekeeping under the foreskin, it's easier for them to make their way up the urinary tract. Therefore, UTI and kidney infections may result in a small minority of cases (1.4 percent, according to Wiswell). The pro-circumcision theory is that removal of the foreskin and the consequent drying up of the glans can reduce the chances of these organisms establishing themselves and getting in the urinary tract. According to the Swedish doctors, circumcision is *at best* a surgical preventive measure for a low-incidence condition easily treated by less drastic measures, a condition created by hospitals in the first place. They recommend that, just after birth, the underforeskin area be deliberately colonized with the mother's intestinal bacteria to prevent UTI. This would certainly be far less drastic than circumcision. Home births address this problem in a different way, as do some hospitals that permit the baby to be in the room with his mother. A lot of physical contact between the mother and child could have a preventative effect on UTIs.

Dr. Wiswell's results have also been challenged on methodological grounds by other physicians. They've objected to the way urine samples were obtained. Wiswell's staff retracted the immature foreskins of the babies, potentially infecting the prepucial space with the germs from their hands, thus inoculating the babies with *E coli*, which covers all our skin and especially our hands.[9]

But supposing for the moment that Wiswell's data is correct, does his recommendation for mass involuntary circumcision follow? Hardly. To cut off a functional body part in order to prevent a low-risk problem is ridiculous.

Another medical doctor, Martin Altschul, did a similar but more methodically strict study of 25,000 baby boys at Kaiser-Permanente Hospitals. A preliminary analysis of his study "...found not a single confirmed case of UTI in a normal male infant. All of the confirmed cases occurred in infants who had clear-cut urinary birth defects."[10]

Another physician, after describing the various problems he deals with, caused by circumcision, goes on to say, "It has been my custom for the last fifteen years to do a routine urinalysis in newborns at two months of age. Rarely is any abnormality found. In fifteen years I have admitted only three infants to a hospital with illness of the urinary tract: two girls with hydronephrosis and a circumcised male with UTI...My experience reinforces the practice of discouraging routine circumcision, a cause of more morbidity than benefit."[11]

So why did Dr. Wiswell get different results? Romberg points out that, although rooming-in status of Wiswell's patients was apparently not recorded, "Kaiser hospitals (from which Altschul got his figures) commonly offer rooming in. Military hospitals (source of the Wiswell studies) frequently do not."[12]

Kaiser Permanente, has a quarterly publication called *Planning for Health.* The Fall, 1995 issue states unequivocally: "Fortunately, urinary tract infections, which are most common among sexually active women under age forty, are easy to treat." In other words, not only are UTIs more successfully treated with much less drastic measures than circumcision, UTIs primarily affect women, not men. And the publication goes on to point out that you can help prevent UTI by simple things like drinking more water.

Penile cancer. Cancer of the penis is a rare disease— with rates around 1 in 100,000 in industrial countries, 1 in 20,000 or 30,000 elsewhere, according to sources cited by Romberg. When it does occur in the U.S., it's usually in an intact man. Penile cancer can usually be treated with partial or complete circumcision if the cancer is inside the foreskin, or with local radiation therapy if on the glans. In extremely rare cases requiring partial amputation of the penis, plastic reconstructive surgery can restore sexual function, something not possible many years ago.

Even if it could be proven that having a foreskin predisposes one slightly to cancer of the penis, that's hardly a reason to cut it off. The chances of serious complications from circumcision are 1 in 500 or 1000, and Dr. Sydney Gellis points out, "There are more deaths each year from circumcision than from cancer of the penis."[13] To put the matter in perspective, we need only note that breast cancer could be prevented by routine mastectomy, yet no one is suggesting routine mastectomy as a preventative.

Phimosis. The inability to retract the adult or late-childhood foreskin because it is too tight and inelastic is called phimosis. The problem usually is treated by American doctors with complete circumcision.

It's perfectly normal for the foreskin to adhere to the glans for the first few years of life, in some cases into the teens or even adulthood. Many well-meaning but uninformed doctors view this normal condition as phimosis and forcefully retract the foreskin or instruct parents to forcefully retract it, tearing it from the glans and leaving the separated skin tissues to grow back together. The more this is done, the more likely that adhering lesions will develop, a condition sometimes called *acquired phimosis*.

So what's the alternative to retracting the foreskin for cleaning? Here's how one physician put it: "One may wash the entire organ [of a child] without attempting to pull back or clean the foreskin. The American Academy of Pediatrics' 1984 brochure on *Care of the Uncircumcised Penis* is good advice to all parents, to all nurses, doctors, and health-care workers. Leave it alone! Let the newborn male take care of his own foreskin when he is able to do it without any trauma or pain."[14]

A foreskin that is too tight can in most cases be remedied by gentle stretching with warm water and creams (soap can cause irritation). In rare cases, a relatively simple surgical slitting of the foreskin—not cutting it off—may be necessary. In even more rare cases, the tip of an inelastic foreskin may need to be removed, but a full circumcision is almost never necessary.

AIDS. Circumcision is now being advocated in the fight against AIDS. One African study is often cited, in which intact men who visited prostitutes in Kenya reportedly showed a higher rate of contamination than circumcised men. Another study [15], however, attributes this to the cultural bias against uncircumcised men, who cannot marry and are more likely to put themselves at risk for AIDS. Questions remain. Why is AIDS in Africa, unlike the West, occurring primarily in the heterosexual population? What are the differences in the strains of the AIDS virus in Africa compared with those in the U.S.? Circumcisionists seem to prefer focusing on Africa, with its many cultural variables, rather than on the U.S., where most men are circumcised and AIDS is widespread, and on Europe, where most men are intact and AIDS, though a serious problem, is less epidemic.

The AIDS-and-circumcision scare tactic apparently started with a letter to the editor of the *New England Journal of Medicine* in 1996 by the late circumcisionist Aaron J. Fink, suggesting a link between AIDS and the presence of the foreskin. The circumcision industry has been trying to find evidence to support this contention ever since.

In rebuttal, Robert Van Howe, M.D. points out that, "While circumcision advocates are quick to cite the small studies that suggest that the foreskin predisposes to HIV-infection, six of the largest studies originating out of Africa have found circumcised men more likely to contract or transmit HIV."[16]

A possible reason why the foreskin would lessen the chances of HIV transmission is that an intact penis can slip gently in and out of its own foreskin during vaginal or anal intercourse. In contrast, a circumcised penis creates more friction and therefore more chance of causing minute tears in the partner's delicate tissues through which HIV can pass into the bloodstream.

And what about the use of condoms, generally recognized as an effective way of stopping the spread of AIDS? Wearing a condom on a circumcised penis has been compared to wearing two condoms on an intact one, since both circumcision and condoms reduce sexual sensitivity. Ironically, mass circumcisions may actually have contributed to the AIDS epidemic in the U.S. by increasing the natural resistance to using condoms. One gay man who was circumcised as an adult wrote:

> ...about 75 percent of my sensitivity was gone...[T]he glans...almost ached for the protection of a warm sheath, which would never be possible again...Concerning anal sex, I was never "big" on it...Now I seek it constantly; it is, in a way, a longing for the protective sheath I have lost—along with its moisture and warmth.[17]

Circumcision simply isn't any sort of "protective shield" against HIV, the virus believed to cause AIDS. Teaching a boy about good hygiene and safe sex will serve him far better. That way, the future option for full sexual pleasure with a safe mate remains. With circumcision, it's diminished forever.

Physicians and medical associations abroad are generally strongly opposed to circumcision. In West Germany, doctors at the Frankfurt Army Medical Center have reportedly refused to perform routine infant circumcisions.[18] Even in Canada, where the practice is still fairly common (though less so than in the U.S.), the Canadian Paediatric Society, reviewing their policy against routine circumcision, concluded, "The present information available concerning the risks of urinary tract infections and transmission of sexually transmitted diseases in relation to circumcision is not sufficiently compelling to justify a change in policy."[19]

While the vast majority of individual doctors in the U.S. do not circumcise, those who do have a great deal of influence. And while medical groups in the U.S. have expressed reservations about circumcision, none have come out in opposition. (The Virginia Urologic Society is a notable exception on the state level.) Why? Romberg believes that, "Many choices in human health care...have centered on who is in control and who is getting paid. A doctor is the person in control when he performs a circumcision. He cannot control whether or not that person is going to wash himself. Similarly, doctors get paid for doing circumcisions, but they do not get paid for telling people to wash." [20]

Yet, it's not just the money. The practice is entrenched in our culture as much as female sexual mutilation is in others.

> "We are aware that there is no medical necessity for this procedure... There would likely be a significant consumer negative response if we refused to perform [circumcisions]... From a marketing and member satisfaction perspective, [we have] elected to continue providing this service to our members. The support for circumcision in this country is cultural and societal, not medical. [We are] responding to societal and cultural expectations by covering this procedure."
>
> —Group Health Cooperative of Madison, Wisconsin [21]

"It has been known for decades that circumcision provides no demonstrably medically necessary purpose. It is rooted in our culture, however."

—Blue Cross Blue Shield of Utah[22]

DR. AARON FINK'S CRUSADE

The late Dr. Aaron J. Fink, a urologist from California, emerged in his retirement years in the 1980s as the most colorful and outspoken of the modern-day circumcisionists. He and his followers denounced preservationists as "foreskin fundamentalists" and "foreskin fanatics." I met Dr. Fink briefly; he seemed to be a sincere and dedicated man. He had become concerned, he told me, when he heard a preservationist doctor give some information on television that he thought inaccurate. He wrote to him, but the reply came instead from the head of the national preservationist organization NOCIRC. Alarmed that there was an actual movement out there—"a network," he called it in a lowered voice, as if it were a dangerous conspiracy—Dr. Fink decided to write and self-publish a book, *Circumcision: A Parent's Decision for Life*, a compilation of historical arguments in support of infant circumcision. He also debated the issue on television, and radio.

Not all urologists share Dr. Fink's point of view. The Virginia Urologic Society in 1986 viewed documentation of a circumcision case that led to "loss of all the skin of the penile shaft" and another that resulted in "gangrene and necrosis of the entire glans and penis due to electrocautery." James L. Snyder, M.D., past President of the Society, was called in for consultation on these two injuries. "I can tell you," he says, "that both of these children will be lifetime genital cripples."[23] As a result of these two cases, the Virginia Urologic Society unanimously passed a resolution against routine infant circumcision.

In his book, Dr. Fink gives four *nonmedical* arguments in favor of circumcision: culture, training, economics, and convenience.[24] Underlying all his arguments is the belief that circumcision doesn't involve any significant loss (though to his credit he does acknowledge it hurts).

Culture. "Parents may wish their son to be like his father or like other boys,"[25] writes Dr. Fink.

According to the American Academy of Pediatrics, "In addition to the medical aspects, other factors will affect the parent's decisions, including aesthetics, religion, cultural attitudes, social pressures, and tradition."[26] Dr. Fink goes farther than the AAP, saying it's okay to circumcise a baby boy for purely cosmetic reasons. This gets to the core of the issue, since the single most common reason parents give for having their sons circumcised is neither health nor religion but simply because they want their son to look like his father or other boys.

The same logic could apply to foot-binding of young girls in pre-revolutionary China and to partial male castration or female genital mutilation as practiced in a number of cultures today. Would Dr. Fink have condoned these practices on similar grounds? When cultural habits are found to be in conflict with biological integrity, which should prevail?

If we look beneath the surface of the expressed concern about a child fitting in, we can often unmask more troubling motivations. The very thought of leaving their sons intact can often be threatening to circumcised men and their mates.

> "What was so difficult in leaving my son intact was not that my son would feel different in a locker room, but that I would feel different from him. I would then have to accept that I'm an amputee from the wars of a past generation."[27]

Most of us never thought to question circumcision, perhaps because it's easier to continue the practice than to face our own loss. We can and should tell our sons, both circumcised and intact, that people used to think the practice was necessary, but now we know better—a simple, truthful, no-nonsense explanation.

Training. In order for the nation to have an ample supply of doctors adequately trained in circumcision, Dr. Fink maintains, we need to keep the circumcision rate up. Listen to the absurdity of that statement. If we didn't routinely circumcise, we wouldn't *need* so many doctors trained to do it.

Economics. Surgery on an adult is more complex because of more bleeding and the necessity of stitches and a separate hospital appointment. It also requires counseling and usually general anesthesia—in short, permission of and consideration for the patient. For these reasons, it's cheaper to cut off the foreskins of all male babies than to remove those of the 5 to 10 percent of boys and men in the U.S. who, Dr. Fink says, will wind up getting circumcisions later in life for one therapeutic reason or another.

Placing monetary value on our body parts is an outrage. Amputating a foreskin as a future cost-cutting measure for the insurance industry is perverse. As an encouraging sign, Medicare in several states and a number of insurance companies have stopped covering routine infant circumcisions, while continuing to pay for therapeutically necessary ones. The state of Washington no longer pays for medically unnecessary circumcision of its employees' children.[28]

U.S. figures for therapeutically "necessary" adult circumcisions are much higher than in Europe. Doctors here tend to think of amputating the foreskin whenever they see even a minor problem. Their European counterparts would be much more likely to try less drastic treatments first.

Convenience. The title of one short subsection of Dr. Fink's book sums up the convenience argument: "Circumcision makes it easy to keep the penis clean."[29] This is a weak argument. Fathers who have been circumcised may have no experience in the very simple practice of cleaning an intact penis, but if a child can learn to wash behind his ears, he can learn to wash his penis.

Even circumcisionists, stop short of the logical implications of their own arguments—mass circumcision of all males, including adults. As Dr. Fink states in his book: "I'm not urging or even encouraging that uncircumcised adult men rush out and have a preventive circumcision. An adult is well aware of his personal hygiene, his sexual habits, and the risk, if any, of his acquiring a sexually transmitted disease. But for a newborn, the case is different. In deciding whether to have a son circumcised, parents are making a choice that may be of great consequence throughout his entire life."[30] What great consequence indeed.

If we were to circumcise even the most slovenly man by force, it would be rightly condemned as a violation of his basic human rights. Yet we accept the same violation of babies' bodies, babies whose future habits we can influence through teaching and personal example.

MEDIA COMPLICITY

Mass media in *any* society tend to report favorably on any information that supports the culture's values and practices. This can be seen in the way our newspapers and magazines print research findings and policy statements on circumcision. The American Academy of Pediatrics' 1989 revision of its long-standing position on circumcision is a case in point. For well over a decade, the AAP maintained the fence-straddling position that "There is no absolute medical indication for routine circumcision of the newborn." Then the organization in 1989 released its long-awaited new position stating that "The procedure has *potential* medical benefits and advantages, as well as *inherent* disadvantages and risks" [emphases mine].

This was little changed from the previous position. If anything, the new statement leaned toward being anti-circumcision, since benefits are "potential," with risks being "inherent" (i.e., certain and unavoidable). AAP President Donald W. Schiff, M.D., said, "We have not reversed our position. We've changed it a bit, but it's really just a bit."[31] Yet newspapers proclaimed this reworded position as a new stand on circumcision. Here are examples of headlines clipped from papers around the country:[32]

"Pediatricians support circumcision: National group abandons previous stand on medical procedure"

"Circumcision policy eased: Doctors' group won't oppose routine practice"

"Pediatricians' statement gives limited approval to circumcision"

"Study backs circumcision to reduce disease"

"Group leans to circumcision: Pediatricians cite possible value"

"Pediatrics group sees benefit in circumcision of newborns"

"Doctors group reverses stance on medical benefits of circumcision"

"Circumcise: Pediatricians say it may not be so bad after all"

"Doctors give ground on circumcision"

"Circumcision: Clear benefits, some risks"

"Academy changes position, calls circumcision beneficial"

"Circumcision again finds favor with doctors"

"Circumcision OK after all, pediatricians' group decides"

As an example of propagandizing, the *Ashbury Park Press* of Neptune, New Jersey received a fairly balanced Associated Press release on the AAP's new position and proceeded to edit out *all* references to disadvantages and risks, headlining the article, "Doctors Find Medical Benefits in Circumcision of Newborns." Anyone reading the article would believe that there were clear benefits and *no* disadvantages or risks.

American Health[33] ran an article in their Family Report section titled "Circumcision's Comeback?" in which it stated that the AAP had "reversed its earlier position" by saying "the procedure 'has potential medical benefits and advantages.'" The full-page article made no mention whatsoever of the "inherent disadvantages and risks" clearly put forth in the AAP statement. It seems that we want science to tell us that what was done to us and what we have done to our children is okay. Here are more items from the actual AAP report:[34]

Meatitis is more common in circumcised boys...

Evidence regarding the relationship of circumcision to sexually transmitted diseases is conflicting.

One study shows...a higher incidence of nonspecific urethritis in circumcised men.

The exact incidence of post-operative complications is not known.

Local anesthesia adds an element of risk.

Infants undergoing circumcision without anesthesia demonstrate physiologic responses *suggesting* they are experiencing pain. [Emphasis mine.]

HEALTH PROFESSIONALS OPPOSED TO CIRCUMCISION

A few pro-circumcision doctors have an undue influence on the policies of medical organizations. In response to this, another group, Doctors Opposed to Circumcision (DOC) has been formed. These doctors are urging the U.S. medical profession to follow other countries that have moved away from the practice of circumcision. There are also prominent U.S. doctors who speak up on TV and radio and through their writings.

Anti-circumcision sentiment is strongest among nurses and midwives. A registered nurse was fired for informing parents of the details of the operation before she obtained the parents' signature on the parental consent form. She later became head of the main anti-circumcision organization in the U.S.

In October 1992, a group of twenty-four nurses at St. Vincent Hospital in Santa Fe, New Mexico, deeply troubled about their participation in circumcisions, refused to assist with them anymore. They were threatened with dismissal, but stood their ground as conscientious objectors to circumcision. Backed by their union, they won. A video has been made about their struggle, *The Nurses of St. Vincent: Saying No to Circumcision.*

> This is not ethical, and especially when you're taking someone who has not consented. *Parents* can consent all they want—that does *not* mean that the *child* has consented!
> —Patricia Worth, R.N.,
> one of the nurses of St. Vincent

In late 1997, Dr. Margaret Somerville, founding director of the McGill Centre for Medicine, Ethics and Law and one of Canada's leading medical ethicists, called the circumcision of baby boys criminal assault and said that doctors should stop doing it.

> It's a wounding, it's clearly a serious wounding—some kids die from this—and the person hasn't given any consent themselves...If you're really looking at something that is traumatic enough that you've got to use anesthetic to do it, should you really be doing that on a newborn baby when it's not needed for his health or health care?[35]

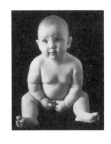

RELIGIOUS BASIS FOR CIRCUMCISION

THE COVENANT BETWEEN GOD AND ABRAHAM

This is my covenant, which ye shall keep, between me and you and thy seed after thee; Every man child among you shall be circumcised.

And ye shall circumcise the flesh of your foreskin; and it shall be a token of the covenant betwixt me and you.

And he that is eight days old shall be circumcised among you, every man child in your generations, he that is born in thy house, or bought with money of any stranger, which is not of thy seed.

He that is born in thy house, and he that is bought with thy money, must needs be circumcised: and my covenant shall be in your flesh for an everlasting covenant.

And the uncircumcised man child whose flesh of his foreskin is not circumcised, that soul shall be cut off from his people; he hath broken my covenant.

—Genesis 17:10–14

Judaism has a tradition of circumcising infants, and Islam of circumcising adolescents. In many Islamic countries, both boys and girls are circumcised, the girls often more severely. Female circumcision, absorbed from African societies into which Islam spread, never had a scriptural basis, but is often considered to have religious significance. Christianity, which started out as a Jewish sect, went through an internal struggle over whether to require circumcision for membership. Perhaps because circumcision would have been a major obstacle for converts to this new, proselytizing religion, the case for circumcision lost. Baptism became the only required ritual, though there are many Christians today who believe circumcision is favored by God because Jesus was circumcised. Baptism may have derived from ancient rites in which priests smeared themselves with the blood of a circumcision or an animal sacrifice, or mixed the blood with water and washed themselves.[1]

MATERNAL INSTINCTS VS. THE COVENANT

The implicit message given to a boy when he is circumcised, whether the ritual is performed when he is seven days old or at puberty, is that your body henceforth belongs to the tribe and not merely to yourself.

—Sam Keen, *Fire in the Belly*

If a woman is made to distrust her most basic instinct to protect her newborn child, what feelings can she ever trust?

—Miriam Pollack
"Circumcision: A Jewish Feminist Perspective,"
*Jewish Women Speak Out:
Expanding the Boundaries of Psychology*

Almost apologetically, I broached the subject of circumcision with a pregnant Jewish friend, whose family had been harassed by the Ku Klux Klan. I knew that criticism of circumcision is often thought to be and sometimes is anti-Semitic.

I was relieved when she thanked me for my concern. As a child, she'd been present at a cousin's *bris millah* (naming ceremony and ritual circumcision). She had been deeply shocked and was very glad she wasn't a boy. "I'd never do that to my child," she told me. "I don't care *who* says I should." An experience in her childbirth classes reinforced her instinctive response:

> One of the parents gave birth early, and we saw the baby. He'd been circumcised, and I watched as she changed his diaper. The end of his penis was so raw, and the urine stung the end of the penis every time he peed. Well, when you're a newborn, you pee all the time! So this poor little kid, what're his first experiences of his penis? For the first part of his life it's all pain. I mean, it must affect him psychologically, and I think his sexuality. I don't see how it couldn't.[2]

My friend's baby turned out to be a boy, and I was invited to a gentle welcoming and naming ceremony in Hebrew and English. There was a party with lots of friends and food, a sort of alternative bris without the surgery. "I'll raise him as a cultural Jew," my friend said proudly of her new son, "and when he's older, the choice will be his."

A small but growing number of American Jews are choosing the option of a *bris shalom*, a naming ceremony of peace rather than surgery. Alternative bris support groups are working to transform the ritual, and increasingly American Jewish boys are going through their bar mitzvahs intact. Circumcision is an open question for the Society of Humanistic

Judaism. The Summer, 1988 issue of *Humanistic Judaism* dealt with the practice in terms of health, civil liberties (infant and body rights), and feminism.

Many Jews are unaware of what circumcision actually is and is not, what it does and does not do, or what it used to consist of compared to what it consists of now. The original form of Jewish infant circumcision removed only the tip of the foreskin, which would have left the penis looking for all intents and purposes uncircumcised to our modern American eyes, accustomed as we are to a more severe "tight" form of circumcision. The switch to this more radical procedure was the rabbinate's response to large numbers of Jewish men practicing foreskin restoration through methods of skin expansion or stretching. Although attempts at getting the foreskin back are probably as old as the practice of cutting it off, for a long time restoration wasn't attempted by enough men to be considered a threat to religious authority. This changed over time, however, in the face of widespread and institutionalized anti-Semitism in Europe. Most recently, during Hitler's reign of terror, when a man's circumcised penis was a death warrant for the entire family, restorative surgery was often attempted.

Circumcising an infant son is not required for him to be considered Jewish. While circumcising an infant son might arguably make a *parent* more observant as a Jew, the child is recognized as Jewish if he has a Jewish mother. Some Reform Jews trace Jewishness through their fathers as well. While being circumcised is often perceived as an essential part of Jewish cultural identity, there are Jewish men—including those born in Europe during the Holocaust who were left intact as a way to help them survive—whose Jewishness is not questioned.

> It is not a sacrament, and any child born of a Jewish mother is a Jew, whether circumcised or not.
>
> —*Encyclopaedia Judaica* (CIRCUMCISION: Laws)[3]

Nonetheless, for Jews the bris is a covenant. For the religiously orthodox, it's a restatement of the covenant between God and Abraham, all of Abraham's descendants and their slaves. For the more humanistic or secular Jew, the covenant is a way of bonding with others who share this ancient tradition. This social and psychological function of the bris is usually strong enough to override the parental concerns of American Jews. The late Edward Wallerstein, author of the book *Circumcision: An American Health Fallacy*, summed up this cultural attachment:

> Having conducted dozens of discussions on this subject, I have found one reaction typical among Jewish physicians. I will paraphrase their comments: "I agree that there are no health benefits. I even feel that it may be wrong to do it. Yet, if I have a son, I will have him circumcised. Please don't ask me why. I am not in the least bit religious. I know it is irrational, but I will do it."[4]

PATRIARCHY AND TRADITION

Despite some indications that in the past women were honored and powerful—for example, Jewishness coming through the mother—Judaism is essentially patriarchal. Circumcision seems to be a patriarchal phenomena, prevalent only in societies in which there are patriarchal groups with a vested interest in the practice—for orthodox Jews, the *mohelim*, for the rest of us in the U.S., the modern priesthood of physicians.

As in other societies, Jewish circumcision probably originated as part of a pre-Hebraic puberty rite, a blood ritual, possibly because men were envious of girls' natural initiation into adulthood through menstruation. The modern-day bar mitzvah may be a remnant of that ancient adolescent circumcision ceremony. Even today, in the rare cases when a Jewish boy is born without a foreskin, blood must still be drawn in the ceremony. In some cultures, this imitation of females is clear. There are Australian aboriginal cultures in which men with subincised penises strap them up to their bellies so they will resemble vaginas. Some reopen the subincision wound from time to time so they, too, can "menstruate."[5]

In his book *Symbolic Wounds: Puberty Rites and the Envious Male*, Bruno Bettelheim argues that with the development of pre-Hebraic culture into monotheism, circumcision was transformed into an infant procedure, reflecting a new power relationship: absolute submission of humans to the new, all-powerful male god.[6] Infant circumcision has to do with social control. If parents can be made—through force, religious injunction, social pressure, or fear of ostracism—to hand over their newborn for mutilation by a medical or religious priesthood, then those parents have fully submitted to the control of that group.

Maimonides had three reasons why infants instead of adolescents should be circumcised: teenagers might not permit the operation, an infant feels less pain, and "...the parents do not as yet love their child with fervent tenderness...For this emotion grows constantly with the sight of the child... Consequently, if circumcision were postponed to the second or third year, it would often be omitted entirely, due to the tender affection of the father for his child."[7]

In fact, genital mutilation is also arguably one useful means to desensitize a boy and socialize him into a culture in which war and other forms of violence are seen to be good or necessary.

Even politically progressive, secular Jews in the U.S. usually have their sons circumcised, though in doing so they often go through rationalizations that to the outside observer seem convoluted. In Harry Brod's anthology *A Mensch Among Men: Explorations in Jewish Masculinity*, the brief chapter on circumcision by Zalman Schachter-Shalomi, a leading rabbi in the Jewish Renewal Movement, quotes such parents struggling with the conflict between protective parental instincts on the one hand and cultural expectations and religious authority on the other. Interestingly, all of the parents given as examples wind up going through with the circumcisions. No mention is made of those Jews in the U.S. and abroad who choose not to circumcise.

The tendency of the fundamentalist aspects of any religious belief system to predominate over a more fluid spirituality is strengthened in the face of external oppression. The retention of cultural practices then becomes an act of courage and resistance, of defiance against the forces of domination. Cultural forms which might otherwise come under criticism and therefore change are reinforced uncritically. To change under threat is to give in to the oppressor. Any form of bigotry or oppression has profound effects on the culture of the target/oppressed group in terms of gender roles, personal self-esteem, and group identification rituals.

And so Jewish ritual circumcision continued secretly under its prohibition throughout history. It's not that the Greeks, the Romans, the Spanish, and others were motivated so much by their concern for helpless infants. They were motivated more by their desire to destroy or control Jewish culture. They may also have been trying to limit the size of the Jewish population, erroneously believing that circumcision enhanced fertility. In the Nazi death camps, circumcision was forbidden. Jews have died rather than abandon this *mitzvah*, and many feel that to give it up now, even just the surgical aspect of it, would be to dishonor their sacrifices.

Holding uncritically to traditional religious forms helps a culture resist external oppression. Yet, as reactive behavior, it also tends to inhibit the expression of spirituality, which is more open, more fluid. When one culture is abused by another, the result is not unlike that of an abused person. Adaptive behaviors and attitudes are developed to help the person or culture survive, but they do not promote growth and happiness, and therefore, outside of the oppressive context, they do not serve the culture or its members positively. To bring something to an illusion of completion, to a final inflexible form, is to have made it finite, and spiritual truth is anything but finite. This seems to be a basic flaw in any fundamentalist form of religion.

The historical impact of anti-Semitism strongly flavors Jewish response to cultural criticism. It also poses serious questions about how Jews can raise the issue of ritual circumcision even among themselves.

> We're members of a Conservative congregation. I remember when we came here, hearing people talk in hushed tones: "Did you know there's a move away from circumcision here in California?" People clicked their tongues in grave disapproval, and fear was in their voices: "It's not good for us." I, too, was shocked. Even now, after the difficult decision not to circumcise our son, we still haven't talked with our rabbi about it because we're afraid he might say he'd rather we weren't part of his congregation.[8]

WHO AM I
TO CRITICIZE?

If it's difficult for Jews to question Jewish circumcision, it's also difficult, in a different way, for a gentile, especially a white, Anglo-Saxon Protestant like me who grew up in the Bible Belt, in the impoverished Ozark Mountain region of north Arkansas. When I walked down the aisle of our old brick church on a Sunday morning one summer long ago, I was followed by others "moved by the spirit." A day and time were set by the preacher, and in a country creek in my best Sunday-go-to-meetin' clothes I was baptized by immersion, soused under the water three times—"In the name of the Father!...and of the Son!...and of the Holy Ghost!" My fellow church members, my beloved community, joyfully sang the old-time hymns on the rocky river bank. The memory is precious to me.

And so I grew up, a small-town boy earning record attendance pins for Sunday school and church with nary a Jew in sight. "We unself-consciously used the expression "to jew (someone) down," meaning "to bargain down," never considering that it might be offensive to someone. I wasn't exposed to the more virulent forms of anti-Semitism until later in life. To my young mind, Jews were biblical characters, along with Pharisees and Sadducees, who existed back in Jesus' time.

When I began writing this book, I was disturbed by the way the preservationist movement had not been able to deal with ritual circumcision, disturbed by statements like, "We're against circumcision except as a religious rite." This seemed to me profoundly dishonest. For if circumcision is what we say it is, and what I feel it in my very flesh to be, then it must be that for everyone who experiences it. It doesn't matter what else it might be, or whatever validation there is for it in one's cultural group. Our bodies are our bodies.

A result of this dishonesty is that some Jewish men have felt not only victimized by their tradition but abandoned by the preservationist movement.

> So much is being done today to educate the public about medical circumcision. However, I see that most of those writing about medical circumcision refuse to discuss religious circumcision. Well, I am twenty-eight years old and have a very unsatisfactory sex life because I lost over half of my glans during a ritual circumcision. Aren't Jewish babies entitled to a foreskin as well? What is really anti-Semitic is the refusal to acknowledge that the

same rights that non-Jewish babies have should be accorded to Jewish babies as well.[9]

I was equally disturbed by some anti-Semitic anti-circumcision writings I had received in the mail after helping to found a group seeking to bring nonviolent direct action into the preservationist movement. Some racist anti-semitic groups rant against circumcision as part of their propaganda. It reminds me of the white-supremacist literature of my native South. One extreme piece of propaganda from such a group combines a few perfectly valid arguments against circumcision with the claim that it causes homosexuality.

> It is unworthy of the advanced White Race to accept such a barbaric practice, just as it is to accept nigger music, nigger and/or Jewish practices, mores, and religions.[10]

There must be, I sensed, some sane alternative to the rationalization of ritual circumcision on the one hand and anti-Semitic tirades on the other. I came to realize that through my involvement in the nonviolent action wings of other social movements I had firsthand experience of a tradition that most active preservationists apparently hadn't, a tradition of dealing with problems of sexism, racism, anti-Semitism, homophobia, or anything else *within* a movement that limits or oppresses its members or others outside it. It seemed to me that, if applied to the preservationist movement, such an approach could open up a space between bigotry and the complicity of silence, allowing for intelligent and heartfelt discussion of ritual circumcision. This sense—and my determination to follow it—has been strengthened by several things during the writing of this book.

First, people in the preservationist movement for the most part seemed not to share my perception that there's a big difference between taking an active stand against anti-Semitism and simply saying, "I'm not anti-Semitic." The latter sounds about as convincing as, "Some of my best friends are Negroes." Even if true, such statements sound suspiciously like a cover for prejudice.

Until fairly recently, people working to end involuntary circumcision feared that if they even mentioned the issues of ritual circumcision, they'd be accused of anti-Semitism. In contrast, a number of friends and fellow activists in the peace and justice movements of the 1980s understood almost immediately the importance of dealing up front with the interconnected and very emotional issues of ritual circumcision and anti-Semitism. And they had the conceptual tools to allow them to deal with such delicate and explosive issues. This led me to believe that the preservationist movement could learn and benefit from such an approach.

Second, in facilitating circumcision workshops, I've found Jewish men to be open to an intelligent reappraisal of ritual circumcision, once they feel it's not just another cover for attacking Jews or Judaism. Of course, men who would come to a circumcision workshop are not by any means a cross-section of society, Jewish or gentile. They are, by and large, men who have already begun to reevaluate a number of beliefs and attitudes. They are also among the ones most able to see both the reality of circumcision and its social and political context. One man in a workshop at the 1989 California Men's Gathering told a very interesting story. While traveling in Africa a few months previously, he had witnessed a female circumcision ceremony and was disturbed by what he felt to be the obvious suffering of the young woman in contrast with the way the tribe was celebrating the event. Upon his return to the States, he was invited to a bris, and was struck by the parallel. Relatives who had been shocked at hearing the female circumcision story were celebrating the cutting off of part of the baby's penis.

Third, the responses to my involvement in this issue by Jewish friends, colleagues, and acquaintances—mostly positive, some defensive, and quite a few a mixture of both—indicate to me that many Jews are undergoing a struggle that's difficult for non-Jews to understand. All except the most defensive have been curious, especially about the hidden history of preservationism within the Jewish Reform movement. Many, especially expectant parents, feel they cannot speak freely of their concerns about circumcision in their own families and communities, and they feel relieved if they give birth to a girl. They feel torn between their cultural heritage and family pressures on the one hand and their own parental instincts on the other. Some suppress their feelings and have their sons circumcised, yielding to tradition. Then, when they see the reality of circumcision, they regret their decision. Still others reject or drift away from the tradition, which they feel puts them in such a bind, just as many felt forced to abandon Judaism in order to marry "outside the faith." One rabbi, who on request will perform a bris without a circumcision, told me that just as Judaism has accommodated the reality of mixed marriages with special programs to allow children to get the best of both parents' traditions, he expected that refusing to let their children be circumcised would be viewed as a valid option by most American Jews within a few decades.[11]

On a personal level, I've chosen to write about ritual Jewish circumcision because it fascinates me. I'm heartened that non-Jews have begun forming a viable preservationist alternative that deals directly and heartfully with the interrelated issues of ritual circumcision, anti-Semitism, and dominator versus egalitarian social relations.

We all have various cultural identities: regional, ethnic, linguistic, professional, social, and political. I call these our tribal identities in the belief that the term "tribal" refers not only to agrarian societies, but also to modern industrial or post-industrial cultures. "American," for example, is a distinctly tribal identity. The view of tribal customs from the outside can be strikingly different than from the inside, and we can often learn from outsiders, as well as from each other. As a white southerner, I'm *glad* that outsiders challenged our practice of racial segregation, which most of us were unable or unwilling to change ourselves. Without outsiders as allies, it is doubtful whether the descendants of former slaves would have been able to overturn legalized segregation. On the other hand, we don't want to judge another culture by the standards of our own and become like missionaries trying to clothe the "naked heathens." So how can we derive the benefits of cross-cultural criticism while minimizing the distortions and chances for abuse? I suggest that when any of us presumes to criticize a practice of another tribe *constructively,* it is important to follow what I call the Principles of Intertribal Criticism.

Principles of Intertribal Criticism

1. Learn about historical and existing rivalries between your tribe and the one being criticized.

2. Learn about past and present disparities in the two tribes' relative political power, as well as in their informal social clout.

3. Clearly define what it is about the practice that you don't like. This prevents your objection to a particular practice from becoming a condemnation of the tribe as a whole.

4. Voice your objections to members of the other tribe, and listen carefully to the responses. Ask questions, but don't argue.

5. Identify the various social and psychological needs that the practice serves for members of the other tribe. Consider other ways in which these needs might be met.

Needs may well be different for different members of the tribe, and the needs of some may conflict with those of others (the male with the female, the rich with the poor, the adult's with the child's, for example).

6. Find out what fears might underlie both the practice in question and any resistance to reevaluating it. Think about ways in which you and your tribe could alleviate those fears.

7. Develop positive personal, political, and/or working relationships with members of the tribe, and find ways to celebrate those aspects of their culture that you like.

8. List the unsavory aspects of your own tribe's history and current practices, both in general and, especially, in relation to the other tribe. Be willing to readily and fully acknowledge these things. In terms of credibility, it is helpful also to have a personal history of speaking out and acting against the unsavory aspects of your own tribe before pontificating about another tribe's shortcomings.

9. Be open to the possibility that you may be wrong, or that you may not have fully understood the context in which the practice occurs.

Ritual circumcision is clearly cultural, and outside criticism of it is cross-cultural criticism, whether or not the practice is defended on other grounds. While circumcision has much deeper cultural roots for Jews, it has become a cultural phenomenon for gentiles, too. Its acceptance by the mainstream U.S. culture indicates just how much we as human beings are capable of coming to view even something that goes against our instincts of self-preservation as normal. To the extent that we can understand Jewish circumcision, we gain insight into how the rest of us have assimilated the practice, as well as how, in the bigger picture, we perpetuate a number of other social, ecological, political, and military practices which are in need of change. Following these Principles of Intertribal Criticism, we can build bridges, dissolve fear, allow each of our various tribes to transcend a parochial view, and learn a good deal from each other.

TAKING PERSONAL
RESPONSIBILITY

In taking a stand against bigotry, we need not become self-righteous, nor should we criticize people with prejudiced attitudes in the same way they criticize others. Neither we nor they are bad people for having prejudicial attitudes learned from others. I have yet to meet anyone who is not prejudiced in some form or another (though it's hard for each of us to see our own biases). In fact, what we call prejudice is often just misinformation, or correct information taken out of context and blown out of proportion—as a person pained over his own circumcision might view Jews as "barbaric" because they circumcise, ignoring the many positive aspects of the culture. This incomplete or distorted view of another group then gets amplified by frustrations and painful experiences in other areas of our lives. We all inherit this stuff in gross or subtle form from others, from our family, friends, and society.

It's fueled by our own frustrations and locked in by our old unhealed traumas. We're not to blame for this; it's not our fault. It doesn't mean we're bad. We are, however, responsible for how we deal with it, what we do with it. Once we're aware, we have a choice: we can continue in our unthinking patterns, or we can discuss our attitudes and behavior openly, exploring the implications and alternatives.

Whether we're talking about circumcision or bigotry, it's essential to find out how we got to where we are and to understand the historical factors behind the cultural behavior. To the extent that we do so, we can stop being slaves of the past and of the powers that be. We can explore alternative ways to achieve whatever positive functions are now served by otherwise destructive behaviors. A fundamental principle of social and cultural change is that for any institution or practice we wish to change, we must identify whatever positive functions it serves in order to find alternative ways to serve those needs. We do have options. It's up to each of us to choose how we manifest our spirituality, in which ways we express and evolve our cultural identity. The responsibility of choice is inescapable. Even if we unquestioningly follow tradition and authority, we are *choosing* to do so. In this age of nuclear overkill and ecological crisis, a serious reevaluation of our ways of thinking and acting would seem to be in order. Whatever serves to create a viable and humane future can be embraced and nurtured. That which does not contribute in this way we can leave rapidly and respectfully behind.

After I left Arkansas and involved myself in the War on Poverty and later in the anti-Vietnam War movement, I gradually came to notice that there was a disproportionate number of Jews among my fellow activists, as has been the case in other social change groups I've been involved in since that time. In his introduction to *A Mensch Among Men: Explorations in Jewish Masculinity*, Harry Brod recounts some of the reasons commonly given for this disproportion: the Jewish "commitment to justice and equality, its messianism, and its emphasis on intellectualism and ideas, and other more sociological factors, such as the particular marginality of Jews, the economic and social roots of anti-Semitism, and a historical sympathy for the underdog." So on the issue of circumcision, it's not surprising that some of the most dedicated preservationists are Jewish men like Edward Wallerstein, author of *Circumcision: An American Health Fallacy*, a major medical work on the subject; Dean Edell, M.D., a nationally syndicated radio and TV medical advisor; publisher Ralph Ginzburg, veteran of free speech battles and Director of O.U.C.H., Inc. (Outlaw Unnecessary Circumcision in Hospitals) in New York; Paul Fleiss, M.D., a pediatrician; Ronald Goldman, Ph.D., author and founder of the Circumcision Resource Center (CRC) and Jewish Associates of the CRC; and feminist educator Miriam Pollack. There are many activists like the one who wrote the following:

> As a Jewish boy, I was circumcised at a religious ceremony. I first found out from some older woman who once

gushed, "Look how big you've grown. I remember you at your *bris!*" That's when I found out not only about circumcision, but that they actually had a party to celebrate, and that strangers were present to watch. I felt a tremendous sense of violation.

I get angry when I hear it classified as elective surgery. From the point of view of the victim, it is no more "elective" than the surgery that Dr. Mengele "elected" to perform on concentration camp inmates.[12]

While it may be tempting to dismiss this statement as trivializing the victims of the Holocaust—or as an example of internalized anti-Semitism—to do so would be to trivialize this man's feelings. The reference to elective surgery goes directly to the core of the issues of infant rights and informed consent of the one affected. The whole statement is a criticism of the trivialization of male genital mutilation.

Because of the history of anti-Semitism, it must be the Jews who lead the fight against Jewish circumcision. The quality of our solidarity in that struggle—and whether it helps or hinders the fight—depends on the extent to which we are willing to confront the anti-Semitism in ourselves and others. The last few years have shown an increased willingness to do this, resulting in less fear and defensiveness all around.

THE JEWISH REFORM MOVEMENT AND CIRCUMCISION

The Jewish Reform Movement started out in the early 1800s as a lay movement—ordinary people taking charge of their social and spiritual heritage. A wide variety of obligations under Talmudic law were reevaluated, changed, or simply dropped. Synagogues became temples, dietary laws went out the window, services were conducted in the national language instead of Hebrew, and so on. Few Jews today have any inkling that for quite a number of years circumcision was dropped altogether in the early Reform movement. Then, as many rabbis took notice of this growing lay movement and became involved in it, many of the initial changes—including the abolition of circumcision—were reversed.[13] Circumcision was not reinstituted without a battle, however. Many people were scathing in their condemnation of the practice. One was

Felix Adler, Columbia University philosophy professor, former rabbinical student, founder-to-be of the Ethical Culture movement, and son of a leading Reform rabbi, Samuel Adler. He viewed circumcision as "simply barbarous in itself and utterly barbarous and contemptible in its origin."[14]

The preservationists eventually lost the battle to an increasingly conservative Reform leadership, and, as a result, circumcision is practiced by most Reform Jews in the U.S. today. It's usually done in a hospital, with a naming ceremony performed separately later. As a result, an intact baby boy can now be taken to a Reform synagogue where the naming ceremony is conducted with the assumption that the circumcision has already taken place. There might even be a rabbi sympathetic to parental reservations about circumcision who will perform the ceremony, no questions asked. A *havurah* rabbi would probably be the best choice, one with an informal meeting group and no official congregation. He or she would have less at stake and be more likely to go along with such a controversial request. Official naming certificates are available from the Society for Humanistic Judaism.

I was quite surprised when, at one synagogue I visited, the office manager compared the clitoridectomies performed on girls in other cultures with male circumcision. "I guess you can tell where I stand on this," she said. "It's genital mutilation."

Of course, such attitudes can be discounted by the orthodox as the corrupting influence of secular humanism. One Jewish man came up to me at an outreach table I was staffing at a university, dismissed humanistic strains in Judaism as fleeting aberrations in the vast panorama of history, and justified circumcision because it was a practice of great antiquity. I pointed out that many Moslems circumcised both boys and girls, and asked, "If tradition and scriptures said to circumcise your daughters, would you do it?"

"No, of course not," he said. "There are limits."

Yesh G'vul—"there are limits"—became the rallying cry and name of the peace movement among Israeli soldiers shocked by their government's actions against the Palestinian *intifada* or uprising. We all have limits beyond which we will or should not go, even under orders of a respected authority, or in pursuit of what we consider to be laudable ends.

What the preservationist movement is doing is drawing the line, the limit, between helpless babies and adults able to make informed choices about their own bodies. In fact, one of the fall-back proposals in the Reform movement as circumcision was reinstituted was to make it an adult procedure, one of free choice, perhaps with only a small portion of the foreskin removed. Unfortunately, it failed.

The issue of circumcision can seem simple, but for Jews its roots go far back into history, as deep as the collective trauma of genocide. When we speak of the pain and loss of circumcision, what many Jews hear is not our compassion or logic, but historical echoes of pogroms, of evictions from ancestral lands, of shattered glass and dreams, of the rap on the door before being taken away. The siege mentality—the

wagon train under attack—that has been created by historical anti-Semitism has made cooperation difficult between
Jews and gentiles with common preservationist aims. Jews
working with gentiles in the movement are sometimes
viewed as consorting with the enemy.

So the issue is far more profound and difficult for Jews
than the mere century-old medical arguments and the
parental insecurities that gentiles have to deal with. For some
reason this seems especially true for Jews in the U.S. The
Summer 1988 issue of the journal *Humanistic Judaism* carried
an article titled "A Mother Questions *Brit Milla*":

> Coming from a European background where routine cir-
> cumcisions as practiced in most American hospitals are
> nonexistent, and where many Jews reject a brit milla as
> an archaic and barbaric ritual, I simply assumed that the
> [American] Jewish community had divergent approaches
> to this issue just as with every other aspect of Judaism. I
> was stunned to realize that questioning this ritual is the
> ultimate taboo among American Jews. Not only was I not
> supposed to question it, but I was not even supposed to
> have the feelings and concerns that I had...Anyone who
> dares to question the brit milla ritual is angrily silenced,
> laughed at, lightly dismissed, or labeled "a traitor under-
> mining Judaism"...[15]

But change is in the air. Feminist Jewish women in Israel
have now carried the Torah to the Wailing Wall and led
prayers there, outraging Orthodox rabbis who seek to pre-
serve unquestioningly the old patriarchal ways. ("A woman
carrying a Torah," *The New York Times* quoted the Orthodox

rabbi in charge of the area as saying, "is like a pig at the Wailing Wall."[16]) The Alternative Bris Support Group (see Resources) is helping the small but growing number of parents who choose not to circumcise while still raising their children as cultural or even religious Jews.

> There is a new public campaign in Israel to ban circumcision. The effort is led by a nonprofit organization whose charter calls for bringing an end "to the primitive act of circumcision." One of the leaders called circumcision "a violent act against the infants." The group distributes literature urging Israelis not to circumcise their sons.[17]

As the Us/Them, Jew/Gentile wall comes down, deep internal value differences between fundamentalist and humanistic Jews emerge. These differences are becoming more and more apparent on a variety of issues, as happened with Israeli policies in the Palestinian uprising. Already we're beginning to see a sort of preservationist version of liberation theology, as some rabbinical students and even rabbis are questioning circumcision, following the lead of lay people. A few courageous Jewish men and women are carrying forward the work of last century's Jewish preservationist movement.

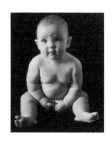

Healing Our Culture, Healing Ourselves

THE LOSS

Both male and female circumcisions raise the same human rights questions. Our mutual fight is against ignorance. People like us, those who have the pain, are the best fighters, because we know the pain of circumcision. What happened to you, you can't change it, but you can help to stop it from happening to other children.

—Shamis Dirir, Coordinator,
London Black Women's Health Action Project[1]

In the U.S., where Jews are less than 3 percent of the population, circumcision is overwhelmingly a secular, not a religious, phenomenon. It's an issue for *all* men in this country, for our sexual partners, and for all those who love us. As men, we're socialized to deny our softer, more nurturing sides. We are often emotionally or physically coerced to do so. In the U.S., most of us are welcomed into life by having part of our penises cut off.

I remember my own post-surgery wailing at age six: "Oh, my penis! Oh, my penis!" My cries, wave after wave of hurt and pain, filled the corridors of the small-town hospital. And I was relatively lucky, mind you. I'd had the benefit of general anesthesia during the surgery. My foreskin had developed lesions to the glans in a way that caused pain in urination, perhaps because it had been prematurely pulled back as doctors frequently and ignorantly do or advise parents to do. A circumcision was recommended to solve the problem once and for all.

My mother decades later regretted not having explored alternatives: "At times my conscience bothers me about having you circumcised. It seemed right at the time to do as the doctor encouraged us. I knew so little about it...I can see so many ways I'd do it differently now." She said that hearing me after the surgery was heart-rending. "You thought you were ruined, for sure!" she recalled, laughing.

Ruined? No. Sex is wonderful for me, but I wonder how much better it might be if all that nerve-laden tissue had not been sliced away. I also wonder how it might be if the doctor had bungled his task. Would I still be able to focus on what I have rather than on what I've lost? One man who was circumcised as an adult wrote: "The acute sensitivity never returned; circumcision destroys a very joyful aspect of the human experience for both males and females."[2]

There are complex psychological factors at work with the loss of erotic tissue like the foreskin and frenulum and with the resultant decrease in sensitivity of the glans. Men circumcised as adults provide a good source of information on how circumcision affects sexuality. Some report a short-term increase in sensitivity before desensitization sets in within a few weeks, months, or, in rare cases, years. Some are happy with their circumcisions because they relieved a medical condition. They usually don't understand that their problem might have been remedied with less drastic measures by a doctor who valued and understood the role of foreskins. Others say they like the lessened sensitivity because it gives them more control over ejaculation. Yet the same circumcision may have a very different effect later on. Desensitization becomes more pronounced as a man grows older, and it can lead to problems in achieving orgasm at all.

It may be that men who were circumcised in adulthood need to justify their post-operative state by focusing on real or imagined positive aspects. A considerable number of such men, however, are not happy with their condition, their feelings ranging from disappointment to depression to intense rage. Some have a mix of feelings. One man in his late fifties wrote to a medical advice column that he had had "a much needed circumcision"—why it was needed he didn't say—but that now he "could not get an erection to have a normal sex life."[3] All too typically, the doctor told him the circumcision probably had nothing to do with it and advised him to explore other causes.

At the First International Symposium on Circumcision, one speaker, who had been circumcised in adulthood, described the difference between pre- and post-operative sexual sensation as akin to seeing a movie in color compared to black and white. The function remains, but certain sensory input simply isn't there anymore.

One circumcised circumcised man I talked to had undergone surgery to have the foreskin restored. He reported a great difference in sensitivity and pleasure between having and not having a foreskin. When he was looking for a competent and sympathetic surgeon, he had been ridiculed. He compared the psychological implications of his foreskin loss with a woman's loss of a breast. "No one today would tell a woman she shouldn't be emotionally traumatized by the loss of part of her body," he says. "It's a natural reaction. So how dare they tell me I shouldn't mourn my loss and want my foreskin back?"

The voices of those who know they've been wounded and are willing to say so are often conspicuously absent from any discussion of circumcision. One of the effects of trauma, especially early trauma, is learned helplessness. If we're subjected to great pain that we have no control over, we learn that life is not only violent, but that the violence is overwhelmingly powerful and disempowering.

The victims of circumcision belie the claim that "the baby gets over it." It's possible, of course, to dismiss such complaints as symptoms of other psychological problems, just as it is possible to write off the psychological dysfunctions caused by racism, sexism, and poverty as purely personal responses. But considering the fact that most circumcised men are denied information about the effects of circumcision, and that there is such strong social validation for the practice, it's quite remarkable that there are any voices of protest at all.

In general, the medical and scientific communities have not considered the psychological impact of genital mutilation important enough to study. What we have instead is anecdotal evidence, a disturbing number of reports from individual victims. Some men, realizing what's been done to them by circumcision (some have carried this knowledge all along), fall into deep mourning. It's natural, as is the reaction to any loss. Activists in the preservationist movement can report numbers of cases of men locked for years into their suffering. Franklin Abbott, psychotherapist and author of *New Men, New Minds: Breaking Male Tradition*, talks about coping with loss:

> Loss and the inability to make it up or make it right can be more frightening than death itself. It can also be a portal to a deeper understanding of self and an invitation to a more radical aliveness. We are challenged by the loss to believe it, to grieve it and to let go of what was true before the loss occurred in order to live authentically in the present…
>
> We do not always choose our losses but we can choose to respond to them bringing to bear our intelligence, intuition and compassion…On the other side of grief are new possibilities, greater wisdom and deeper loving self-acceptance. In nature fires are necessary to keep forests and swamps vital ecosystems. Though it may not be your lightening that has ignited the fire that created the loss, how you live with it, day by day, hour by hour, is largely up to you.[4]

MASKING
THE MUTILATION

The anti-circumcision movement for decades has emphasized the pain the baby feels as the main reason that circumcision should stop. However, the focusing on pain has proved to be a weak strategy. It has given circumcisionists the incentive to counter this concern by developing more effective anesthetics for use in circumcisions. These products will be coming on the medical market in the coming years. By lessening the immediate trauma of the operation, circumcisionists sidestep questions of body rights and the long-term effects of circumcision.

The first piece of circumcision pain-management legislation in the country has been introduced into the Michigan state legislature, which "...forbids physicians to perform surgery on any child who is strapped in the circumcision restraint board and not given anesthesia...[and] mandates that parents be fully informed about the availability and risks of pain management before consenting to the procedure. It states that health-care providers must be trained and continuously updated about pediatric pain management."[5]

Note that this wording allows for a baby to be circumcised without anesthesia if he's not strapped into a circumcision restraint board, and that his parents can still consent to unanesthetized circumcision. While health-care providers must be trained in pain management, there's no mention of educating them about the human rights issues involved in circumcision.

The language in the Michigan bill is derived from federal guidelines for the use of animals in invasive and painful research. Such "humane" guidelines seek to decrease the suffering of some of the animals (many are exempt, depending on their species and whether the experiment would be compromised by use of pain management techniques). These "humane" guidelines help quiet public outrage over abuses.

Many health professionals have supported the Michigan legislation, which came about because one nurse, appalled at the suffering she witnessed year after year, approached her state senator, who collected co-sponsors and introduced the bill despite opposition from influential doctors.

> We do not have the moral luxury to permit physician-inflicted pain to continue during our ongoing battle against circumcision.[6]   —Nancy Mulnix, R.N.

There is a difference between working for reforms versus working for abolition of a problem. Facing the horrors of slavery in the U.S., for example, some white people put their efforts into passing laws requiring owners to treat slaves better, while others put their efforts into the abolition of slavery. Some preservationists divide their energies between reform and abolition, and working for reform can lead to abolition.

I remember once going to hear Helen Caldicott, past president of Physicians for Social Responsibility. After her rousing talk on the dangers of the nuclear arms race, someone in the audience asked, "What can I do? What group can I join?" Dr. Caldicott refused to tell her what she should do. "You have to follow your heart, find the areas of work that call you and ways of working that work for you, instead of following somebody else's idea of what you should do." The same is true for the preservationist movement. By following the "right" way for you, the way your own heart and mind lead, you will have more energy and clarity for the work. A strength of the preservationist movement is the diversity of its approaches to the problem.

We have a limited amount of time and life energy, and we must choose where we put our efforts. Putting them in one area means they can't be put in another. If we put our efforts into reform like pain management of circumcision, it's important to make sure that this is a first step toward abolition. We must say this loud and clear and keep saying so. Otherwise our efforts may have the unintentional effect of causing parents and the public to become acquiescent again on the issue.

In Italy, faced with the female sexual mutilation practiced by some immigrants, the health authorities decided to circumcise the girls in state hospitals, less severely and under anesthesia. France and England decided instead to use child abuse laws to prohibit the procedure. Which course do we take? How much weight do we give to the pain, how much to the mutilation? These are questions that the preservationist movement and children's rights advocates will have to answer.

> ...all anesthesia does is mask the pain. Unfortunately, anesthesia will never mask the mutilation—that will always be there."

> —Tim Hammond
> Founder, National Organization to Halt the
> Routine Mutilation of Males (NOHARMM)

FORESKIN RESTORATION

Foreskin restoration is now becoming a mainstream issue as evidenced by this excerpt from "Sex Matters," a newspaper advice column written by Louanne Cole Weston, Ph.D.:

CIRCUMCISED MEN WANT IT ALL BACK

Q: My husband of many years recently expressed his feelings of anger and loss at the fact that he was circumcised as a baby. He says that it was a totally unnecessary and senseless surgery that has deprived him of protection for the head of his penis and undoubtedly caused him to lose some sensation, not to mention that it was done entirely without his knowledge or consent!

More recently he told me he had found some information on the Internet about foreskin restoration which involves taping and stretching the remaining skin to form a kind of substitute foreskin. He has started to do that. Based on the experience of others who have done this, he says that the process may take a year or more to produce significant results. Obviously, he cannot recover what was cut off from him so long ago, but he says that it will be worthwhile if it makes him feel better and if he does regain some sensitivity.

Is this a sign of male menopause or what? As far as I can determine he has very adequate sensitivity and has never experienced any kind of problem that I am aware of. I have even offered to knit him a cap to wear over the head of his penis but he has said no thanks to my idea. Furthermore, I do not particularly care for the appearance of uncircumcised penises.

Is this something I should just chuckle about quietly and allow to run its normal course, hoping he tires of the daily taping routine? Or might it produce some real benefits for him? Are significant numbers of other men also trying to return to their natural glory? Or is this an isolated case?

A: Your husband is actually part of a growing number of men who as adults are questioning a surgical procedure that was routinely performed on most infant males for several decades in the U.S. And now he and they are doing something about it.

Fortunately (in my opinion), many parents, physicians and nurses no longer allow the often unanesthetized cutting away of such highly sensitive skin and tissues. Down from its peak level of 85 percent in 1980, circumcision occurred for about 63 percent of infant boys in the U.S. in 1994. According to the National Center for Health Statistics, parents on both coasts have dropped the practice more quickly than in the Midwest, with the West showing a rate of 34 percent circumcising in 1994.

The technique your husband is using to restore the protective function of his former foreskin has been practiced for several years. For more information on the whys and how-tos, read: *The Joy of Uncircumcising! Restore Your Birthright and Maximize Sexual Pleasure*, by Jim Bigelow (Hourglass Book Publishing, 1992).

Many men who were circumcised as infants have a hunch that the skin on the head of the penis has changed. If they made comparisons with an uncircumcised man they would see and feel the difference, a thickening of the skin. The cap you proposed knitting would need to be made of slightly moist skin and would only be removed during bathing and sexual activity to accomplish its task. Otherwise, it is no different from the rubbing against clothing an uncircumcised man typically experiences.

...You mentioned that you do not care for the look of intact penises. Should the aesthetics of genitals be reason enough to cut parts off? I do not think so. Most women would not want men surgically redesigning their external genitals—although unfortunately that does go on in certain parts of the world.[7]

They are coming back in droves, those who were circumcised, wishing to be uncircumcised. Many are intelligent individuals. They are challenging our primitive habits and attempting to elevate us out of the ignorance of the past.

—Anthony Orlanndella, M.D.[8]

Like the great majority of men my age in the U.S.—including doctors who circumcise and judges who preside over legal challenges to the practice—I don't really know what I'm missing. I can't.

All, however, is not lost. While the skin, nerves, and blood vessels of my former foreskin and frenulum are gone forever, it is possible to once again have a foreskin. How? There are two ways: surgery and the prolonged stretching of remaining skin. Both these techniques are ancient and both have been improved. Surgery is far quicker, with immediate results after a short period of recuperation. It's expensive, though insurance companies sometimes pay. It's also riskier—you may wind up with an inadequate or botched restoration job and be worse off than before. One man I met had spent some time with skin expansion techniques with good results, but was impatient. He researched restoration surgery, found doctors who would do it (there are very few), and interviewed both the doctors and their former patients. He was so happy with the results of the procedure that he could hardly stop talking about his increased pleasure and newfound sense of wholeness. He, however, recommended that men first try the more gentle skin expansion techniques before considering surgery, and that surgery should not be undertaken without thorough research.

Skin expansion is based on a simple principle. When skin is stretched, the stretching causes microscopic tears between the skin cells. If the stretched skin is released, as is usually the case, it returns to its prior condition. However, if the stretching is constant—as with the skin of a person gaining weight—the body manufactures new cells to fill in between the separated ones. This results in new skin.

The most common technique is to stretch the remaining foreskin (or, if there isn't any, the penis's shaft skin) and tape it in the stretched position. Circumcised men with some remaining foreskin will be able to get a new foreskin in less time than required by men with "tight" circumcisions, still, it's not quick. The time usually required is two to four years of fairly consistent stretching, depending on the amount of skin left, the elasticity of that skin, how consistent you are in stretching, whether you leave the stretching device on at night, and so on. I used a taping technique just during the daytime for a number of months until international travel and a reactivated sex life distracted me from my efforts. During the time I did do it, I was surprised by how much better I felt having my glans covered by my own natural skin, something I'd lived my whole adult life without experiencing.

Quite a few men give up before completing this process. Some of those resume it later, as I may well do. Those who see it through to completion report that the effort is well worth it. In a workshop I helped facilitate at a California Men's Gathering, was another facilitator who had been doing the skin expansion technique for some time. As the workshop ended, he agreed to show the results of his foreskin stretching to anyone who was interested in staying after. Needless to say, he stole the show. Nobody left, and everyone—myself included—was astounded at the full foreskin this man had achieved through a simple stretching technique he had developed himself.

Skin expansion techniques are medically recognized, but doctors are not yet prescribing them for foreskin growth, perhaps because they wouldn't make money on it, perhaps because they think the goal is a trivial one, perhaps because the patient, not the doctor, is in control of the process.

According to an article in *Sex Life* magazine, an estimated 7,000 to 10,000 men in the U.S. are currently undergoing foreskin restoration.[9] Support groups have formed to help men through the process, and books like *The Joy of Uncircumcising* by Jim Bigelow tell in detail just how to do it. (See Resources.)

INFANT RIGHTS

Circumcision boils down to a matter of personal and cultural choice, but—and this is crucial—*it should be the personal and cultural choice of the one being circumcised*. We men have as much right to control our bodies as women do theirs, a right that in the U.S. is routinely violated with infant circumcision.

The Articles of Convention of the International Save the Children Fund places that organization "against all forms of physical and mental injury to children."[10] The pain, the loss, and the risk resulting from circumcision are in violation of Article 5 of the Universal Declaration of Human Rights, adopted by the United Nations General Assembly on December 10, 1948, and binding on all member states, including the U.S.:

> No one shall be subjected to torture or to cruel, inhuman or degrading treatment...

And UN Resolution 44/25 of 1989, Convention on the Rights of the Child, states explicitly in article 24 section 3:

> Parties shall take all effective and appropriate measures with a view to abolishing traditional practices prejudicial to the health of children.

If not for our cultural bias, we would see that cutting off part of a baby's genitals is "cruel treatment." But it's not likely that either the Save the Children Fund or the United Nations will come out against male infant circumcision. A number of member states including the U.S. consider the practice culturally and religiously sacrosanct. There is a ray of hope, however. The UN in recent years, despite accusations of "cultural imperialism," has begun to address the more extreme forms of female circumcision.

LEGAL ACTIONS

Several cases have been brought in U.S. courts, including one by a rabbi's wife against the *mohel* (Jewish ritual circumciser) who circumcised her son against her will, and another on behalf of a baby boy who was circumcised without his mother being adequately informed about the operation before signing the consent form. Legal issues include battery, false imprisonment, sexual assault, child abuse (a "nonaccidental physical injury"), informed consent (whether the parent has been adequately informed about the procedure before giving their consent), and infant rights (whether the parent even has the right to consent to surgery on a baby who has no medical problem that requires it).

In Britain, a four-year-old Muslim boy was awarded £10,000 (about $17,000) provisional damages from the rabbi who botched his circumcision, necessitating three corrective surgeries. The court said the award would be later increased if the boy developed psychological or sexual problems after puberty.[11]

And in the Fall/Winter 1995 issue of the NOCIRC Newsletter, the following cases were reported in the "Legal Action" column:

- An eight-year-old Russian Jewish immigrant boy received an out-of-court settlement of $1,200,000 from a clinic in Brooklyn for a circumcision performed by a doctor and a rabbi in which the boy lost part of the head of his penis.

- In Houston, Texas, in 1995 a five-year-old boy went into a coma while being circumcised and died a week later.

- $256,000 was awarded to a boy who lost a third of his glans in a circumcision at a Navy hospital.

- $65,000 in damages was awarded to a boy circumcised in 1995 at Jackson Hospital, Montgomery, Alabama, without his parents' consent.

- $36,400 was awarded to a boy in San Diego, California, whose glans was cut off during his circumcision in 1992.

- A urologist in Vancouver, Canada was ordered to pay $40,000 in damages to a man who required surgery to repair damages done when he was circumcised at age twelve.

In addition, the newsletter reported the case of a boy who in 1986 was circumcised the day after he was born at Providence Hospital in Anchorage, Alaska. He developed complications and went into a prolonged seizure or "crash" which left him severely brain damaged and unable to walk, talk, or care for himself in any way. His parents were offering $10,000 as a reward for information leading to the recovery of missing medical records covering the critical 26-hour period prior to his seizure.

Preservationist organizations have not had the funds for well-researched cases and multiple appeals, and so no high-level precedent has yet been set that would protect baby boys. It's not surprising that U.S. courts have restricted their concern to accidents occurring during circumcision, ignoring the legal issues raised by the procedure itself. They have been reluctant to rule in favor of male infants' fundamental right to their genitals, for to do so would be to make criminals out of doctors. It would also raise politically explosive issues of religious freedom and separation of church and state. And the courts are no more willing to apply international law (such as the Universal Declaration of Human Rights cited above) to the practice of genital mutilation than they are to hear challenges to the policy of nuclear deterrence, which, as a threat of "mass and indiscriminate destruction" of civilian populations, is also illegal under international law.

Courts are seldom willing to buck entrenched social prejudices, but we can find encouragement from looking at the history of other modern social reform movements. As the social and political climate around this issue continues to change—through education and outreach as well as more dramatic acts of public protest and civil disobedience—we can expect that legal decisions will continue to shift. What is now controversial—the idea that babies' genitals should be left in their natural state—will then seem obvious, and people will be astonished that we used to do such a thing to our children.

> "All truth passes through three stages. First, it is ridiculed. Second, it is violently opposed. Third, it is accepted as being self-evident."
>
> —Arthur Schopenhauer

DIRECT ACTION

U.S. Doctors debate circumcision endlessly, just as the arguments went on and on in my native South about whether blacks had the same mental capacity as whites, and whether segregated black schools were as good as the white schools. While it was necessary to engage in such debates in order to expose the misinformation that supported institutionalized oppression, it was black people and white allies finally standing up, marching, sitting in, and saying: "No more!" that sent Jim Crow reeling. It was Stonewall that launched gay rights into the political arena, and street demonstrations and draft resistance that helped extract us from Vietnam.

Action speaks louder than words, but the two together are even more powerful. Those of us victimized in various ways and to varying degrees by circumcision have a unique power to help parents and policymakers understand that it's not just an academic debate. Some of us have begun to translate our pain and anger into social and political action beyond educational and lobbying work.

> The greatest disadvantage of circumcision, in my view, is the awful loss of sensitivity when the foreskin is removed...I was deprived of my foreskin when I was twenty-six...Really—and I mean this in all seriousness—if American men who were circumcised at birth could know the deprivation of pleasure that they would experience, they would storm the hospitals and not permit their sons to undergo this unnecessary loss.[12]

"Storming the hospitals" has begun. Demonstrations have been mounted at a number of circumcising facilities and outside the headquarters of the company that makes the *Circumstraint*—the board that babies are strapped to for circumcision. At Cornell University Hospital a man was arrested on his second attempt to "retire" a *Circumstraint* board. In his defense, "Baby Boy," as he identified himself, said, "I did steal something from them, but they stole something from me twenty years ago." He was found guilty and sentenced to community service.

Such actions, including those on a larger scale, were the idea behind The Victims Speak, which I co-founded in 1988 (it was later succeeded by the National Organization to Halt the Abuse and Routine Mutilation of Males, NOHARMM). Our founding principles and goals were:

Nonviolence. [We seek] to bring the principles and techniques of nonviolent action...into the [preservationist] movement, giving creative voice to the victims of circumcision.

Culture. We view circumcision as...a cultural phenomena, whether practiced with a medical or a religious rationale and whether performed on infants or adolescents, males or females.

Anti-Semitism. We seek to deal directly with...anti-Semitism, both historically and now—within ourselves, within the [preservationist] movement, and in society at large...

Abolition. We seek the end of all forms of involuntary genital mutilation for whatever reason. We believe that each person has a fundamental right to a gentle infancy, an intact body, and full adult sexuality regardless of race, gender, or parents' belief system.

Unity. We are feminist...*and* we embrace men's rights, seeing no inherent contradiction...We support cultural diversity and those aspects of any philosophy or belief system which unite us in caring relationship to each other and to our bleeding planet.[13]

Solidarity with the women's movement on this issue has been strained by the silence of the major feminist organizations on the issue of male circumcision, while some feminists have been actively hostile. At one film showing and forum I attended on female circumcision in Africa, it was announced at the outset that no discussion at all of male circumcision would be permitted. By doing so, the facilitator, I felt, crippled the ability of the gathering to understand the social and psychological process through which a culture comes to accept sexual mutilations. I got up and started to walk out, only to be booed and heckled by some of the women in the mostly female audience. A friend of mine, a man with extensive organizing experience around women's issues and gay rights, was devastated for months after something similar happened to him. Still, as much as it hurts, it's important to work through such hostility so that we can *all* be heard. My pain doesn't invalidate yours, and yours doesn't invalidate mine.

The task of breaking through the ignorance, habit, and vested interests that support involuntary circumcision has so far fallen upon a few individuals and groups deeply committed to the cause. They pressure hospitals to inform expectant parents about options and risks before they sign the consent form for circumcision, they press insurance companies to stop paying for nontherapeutic circumcisions, they educate expecting parents, and they work for change within their professional organizations. The National Organization of Circumcision Information Resource Centers (NOCIRC) is the clearinghouse for such activism. Its executive director, Marilyn Fayre Milos, R.N., is mother of three circumcised boys and grandmother of one intact child. "We're learning!" she says, laughing. When she's asked about her sons' circumcisions, her sadness comes to the surface. Like many parents, she didn't know any better. She thought it was the best thing to do, that the doctor knew best.

Milos was launched into this cause when, after her children were grown, she decided to become a nurse-midwife. In nursing school she witnessed a circumcision for the first time and was deeply shocked. (Her account of that experience appears at the end of the subsection on female mutilation.) When she was later fired from the hospital for informing parents about the risks of circumcision, she and others founded the non-profit educational organization that later became NOCIRC. Milos is frequently a guest on TV and radio shows around the country, and her regional nurses' association awarded her its highest award for Clinical Excellence in Perinatal Nursing for "almost singlehandedly rais[ing] public consciousness about America's most unnecessary surgery" and for her "dedication and unwavering commitment to 'righting a wrong'..."[14]

Like a number of newer social movements—Green, feminist, gay rights, animal liberation—the preservationist cause has formed outside the traditional political left. It's also been essentially ignored by it. Even books dealing extensively with female circumcision abroad, books like Mary Daly's *Gyn Ecology: The Metaphysics of Radical Feminism*, somehow avoid any mention of the involuntary genital mutilation of male babies in the U.S. This brings up serious questions of cultural or gender bias. While the focus of such books is quite properly on females, are we to assume that the violent and patriarchal nature of infant male circumcision is irrelevant to women's oppression? On another level, are we to believe that the existence of more severe forms or degrees of violation is sufficient reason to ignore lesser forms or degrees? If so, are we then to believe that the existence of rape is a valid reason to ignore mugging, of murder to ignore rape, and of genocide to ignore discrimination? I fail to see the logic that the usually greater degree of mutilation of female children in other cultures somehow makes it okay to mutilate the genitals of male children in our own. Some women, including some feminists, when presented with real emotions and rational arguments against infant male circumcision, react with something like, "Oh, God, there go those men talking about their penises again. Can't they think of anything else?" This trivializes and discounts our personal feelings, experiences, and concerns just as men so frequently trivialize women's concerns. While such attitudes are understandable in the light of women's experience with male violence and desensitization, they nonetheless impede the possibility of a common front against the various violations that both men and women experience.

So why haven't many self-professed progressive organizations in the U.S. endorsed the right of males to have intact genitalia and full, natural sexuality?

- As members of this society, we are all indoctrinated with the desirability or at least the acceptability of male circumcision. It seems normal to most of us, including those who have studied other forms of violence and social oppression. The idea of a man's right to intact genitals may seem foreign and ridiculous to the same people who are outraged at the thought of even the mildest forms of female sexual mutilation.

- In our culture male pain and loss are downplayed if not downright trivialized. Men are sent to war routinely, while the thought of women in battle is troubling. The image of a man being struck by a larger man in a movie isn't nearly as shocking to us as the sight of the same thing happening to a woman.

- A lot of women don't want to hear men "whine" about themselves and their penises—they may be tired of men dominating conversations, they may have been abused by men, or they may simply lack the understanding that men get hurt, too, in ways that women don't.

- The movement against female sexual mutilation emphasizes the severest forms, leaving the impression that all female circumcision is that severe and allowing male circumcision as we in the U.S. know it to be dismissed as much less serious in comparison.

- It's seen as not politically expedient or "feasible" to include males in legislative attempts to protect females from sexual mutilations. It's far easier to rally opposition to the "foreign" practice of female sexual mutilation than to our entrenched, home-grown practice of male sexual mutilation. And there's less chance of alienating potential supporters, creating divisions within their organizations, and/or being labeled anti-Semitic.

As Alice Walker said on National Public Radio: "I think it is a mutilation. I guess in working with female genital mutilation, we often find that the battle is such an uphill one, that we hope that the men who are working on this issue about male circumcision will carry that."[15] If it's an uphill battle to get female sexual mutilation banned, it's an intergalactic war to get our own culture to stop our own sexual mutilation of males. The movement against male circumcision has long expressed its opposition to the mutilation of *all* children, boys and girls. Unfortunately, this solidarity has not been reciprocated.

The strategy of dissociating themselves from male circumcision—whether by dismissing it as trivial or by leaving it up to the men—has been a prerequisite for many activists in making headway against female circumcision, just as many white workers thought dissociating themselves from black slaves to be a prerequisite for "respectability" when they were organizing the unions before the Civil War.

In 1995, the state of North Dakota became the first state to pass a law against genital mutilation—specifically, against female genital mutilation. Other states were soon to follow. What the media *didn't* report is that the drafters of the legislation wrote the bill originally with gender-neutral language that would have outlawed *all* forms of genital mutilation, male and female, but they couldn't get enough support in the state legislature to pass it. When they reluctantly changed the wording to protect females only, legislators eagerly signed on, and the bill passed easily. The drafters themselves have now filed suit against the state claiming that the new law is unconstitutional because it unfairly excludes members of one gender from protection, while all members of the other gender are protected from even the "mildest" forms of genital alteration.

When a speaker from Islamic Africa at the First International Symposium on Circumcision was asked what the revolutionary movements' positions were on the various female and male genital mutilations common there, he replied that because they were fighting for "political," not "cultural," change, these movements took no stand.[16] In terms of male genital mutilation, the same can be said for almost every single labor, liberal, or left-wing group in the U.S. A major alternative publisher of books on peace, justice, and nonviolent social change wouldn't even consider publishing this book (back when it was just an idea), because the subject was too much "on the fringe."

I have often wondered, will our bodies, our genitals, continue to be of no concern to progressives so locked into their traditional agenda and so concerned with being acceptable to their established constituencies? Or will we see an opening of minds and hearts, a restructuring of the way we view culture, our bodies, and sexuality? At present, it's the preservationist movement alone—with virtually no support from anywhere on the political spectrum—that is working to end the American practice of genital mutilation.

Like green/ecology concerns, the preservationist movement is "neither right nor left." It tries to bring out the best of
both progressives and conservatives. It seeks to liberate us
from socially entrenched violence and oppression, and to pre-
serve or conserve that which is good and natural from unwar-
ranted meddling and destruction.

> It is not easy to see evil in something that has the sanc-
> tion of long tradition, but traditions can be bad as well as
> good. They represent inherited error as well as inherited
> truth, and it is the reformer's job to tackle and clear away
> whatever is harmful in them.
>
> —Archbishop Lang (UK)[17]

VOICING OUR PAIN:
ON THE PATH TO HEALING

Silence as a respite from the incessant chatter of the outside world and of our minds is a beautiful thing. Silence about things that need to be said is another matter, reinforcing old ways and inhibiting the advent of better ways of thinking and being. Our cultural silence about circumcision is of the latter sort. As we get in touch with repressed feelings and work through them, we break the silence, we begin to end our complicity. As men apply skin expansion techniques as well as surgical options for foreskin restoration, we not only start to regain a sense of wholeness and sensitivity, we also make a powerful political and cultural statement. The sexual mutilation industry is able to continue because its infant victims are powerless and because we adults passively and silently accept the consequences of what's been done to us.

Breaking that silence is a major step toward abolition. Doing what we can to get back what was taken away from us is an important part of the process. But coming to terms with our psycho-sexual wounding and organizing around the issue can be difficult.

> Many men don't know—and don't want to know—that they've been scarred, that they've been desensitized, that there may be other complications in their sex life.
>
> —Norm Cohen, son of a rabbi

Those who do know they have been scarred are understandably reluctant to acknowledge their loss even among friends, much less to stand up in public and say so. I remember one man who asked to be removed from a contact list for preservationist actions because, he said, "It's too painful for me to be reminded of circumcision in any way." At least he is aware of his trauma. There are many more men circumcised as infants who are in a state of profound denial reinforced by not only a lack of accurate information but also by outright misinformation.

Awareness about circumcision seems much higher among gay and bisexual men, probably because they experience other men's penises and can compare. Most of us heterosexual men never get that opportunity, and we're too inhibited to seek it out. And so we muddle through our sex lives not knowing what we're missing, with no idea of how much better it could be, how we've been ripped off. Had I not met and become friends with an active preservationist, I would have stayed like the overwhelming majority of people in the U.S., uninformed or in denial.

Just as others helped me become aware, this book, I hope, will cause other men to become aware. It's not comfortable knowing that what I write will make others re-experience a violation they've long ago repressed, to comprehend a loss they've been unaware of. It's a responsibility I don't take lightly. Part of me thinks, "It's too late for me, why bother dealing with it?" But another part isn't satisfied, doesn't want to live in denial and, through silence, pass on lies. I don't know of any other way to bring about personal and social healing than for those of us who've been violated to face our denial, to mourn our loss, and then to accept it and to resolve that we shall pass on a better way to our children.

On my forty-third birthday, I was at an all-day dance workshop in an old former church, now a community center, in north London. At one point toward the end of the day, all forty-odd participants gathered in a large circle sitting on the floor or standing, dwarfed by the hall's vaulting ceiling of massive timbers. Someone started humming, and soon everybody was doing it. The different voices, the wordless soundings, became increasingly varied. Mine and my partner's became wailings of unspoken hurts from deep within our breasts. For me, the hurt was the mutilation of circumcision.

Words are so inadequate to express what many of us have to express how we have been violated. To use speech, no matter how eloquently, is to betray the depth of our violation, to betray feelings which don't fit the niceties of conventional speech. We need something deeper. Traditionally, in a variety of social movements, civil disobedience has come from this realization about the inadequacies of speech alone. As Thoreau put it, civil disobedience is voting with one's whole body, not just a slip of paper.

For centuries, people have expressed deep sorrow by keening—a wailing, a wordless cry, a lamentation. That's exactly what we were doing, in that old London church. There could be no more appropriate form of voicing our feelings about what's been done to us. Perhaps through hearing our keening, those who support circumcision will have their hearts opened at last.

I arrived one day at the office of the National Organization of Circumcision Information Resource Centers (NOCIRC) to find its director weeping at the phone. She had just retrieved messages from her answering machine. A brand-new father had called twice while she was out, saying that he and his wife had considered the pros and cons, including a piece of NOCIRC literature they'd somehow come across, and had decided to circumcise. The deciding factor, he said, was that the NOCIRC brochure was "emotional," and so his infant son was set to become, thirty minutes after the last call and in the father's words, "civilized."

We suffer from a tyranny of the intellect over the emotions. A dictatorship of the head over the heart instead of an integration of the two. Tradition dictating to, not being informed by, protective and nurturing instinct. A separation of ourselves from nature, from nonhuman animals, from "uncivilized" peoples. This seems to me a fundamental "dis-ease" at the root of many of our problems, from widespread genital mutilation to class exploitation to sexual violence to nuclear overkill in disguise as national defense. Like so many of the crucial issues we face today, circumcision is highly emotional *and* requires clear-headed thinking and analysis. We need to bring our heads and our hearts together in order to transform our pain and our loss into constructive, effective action.

It took me a long time to begin the process of getting in touch with my suppressed trauma, the grief, the loss that I, like so many men, have experienced. I still can't bring myself to watch a video of a circumcision from beginning to end. The pain is simply too great.

When I tried foreskin restoration, I was surprised at the positive psychological effect I experienced as my penis started to look, to feel, to *be* whole again. In addition to the personal benefit, as more and more of us strive to get back as much as we can of what we've lost, we create a statement against mutilation more powerful than the most eloquent speech. I'm interested in but wary of surgical techniques; even though some insurance companies will pay for the procedure, I have little trust in the profession that cut it off in the first place. I speak openly about the issue with friends and colleagues, and find sympathetic understanding, positive support, and appreciation at least as frequently as joking, aversion, and retreat into tradition (our typically human reactions to uncomfortable new information).

I enjoy the much-needed lightness that humor brings to the subject, though it's sometimes tricky to keep from trivializing the issue in the process. At various times, I've written, facilitated workshops, and helped organize political action against involuntary circumcision. I dream of 10,000 men all across the country, joined by other mutilated men and women all over the world, no longer silent, keening our loss to those who continue to cut off parts of babies' genitals, placing our bodies between the circumcisers and their intended victims, demanding that the violence stop with us, declaring that the healing shall now begin.

One foot in front of the other, this journey has begun. I don't know where it will lead. I only know I have to go.

AFTERWORD

Many of us have been circumcised because our parents thought it was best for us. We've had our sons circumcised for the same reason. We didn't understand the risks. We didn't know about the loss of sexual feeling. We didn't realize that medical reasons for circumcision are attempts to justify a very ancient practice that has outlived whatever useful purpose it may once have had.

Now that we know better, we can begin to allow our children their full biological heritage.

A friend used to take long winter trips to Mexico for his health. In the midst of feeling overwhelmed by the sorting, packing, and planning beforehand, he'd get to a point where he'd simply lock up and go. "If the Captain waited 'til everything was all shipshape before setting sail," he'd say, "the ship would never leave port."

I feel a bit that way about this book. I want to learn more, and I want to find better ways to write and organize what I have to say. In short, I'm still learning, still grappling with the issue and how to present it. On some level, this book will probably never be finished. There will always be some new fact or perspective to be included. But the time has come to put it into the world—into your hands, your head, and your heart—with all its imperfections. If I have offended, whether unnecessarily or by speaking a painful truth, I ask that you let me know. If I have said anything that you feel is unfairly exaggerated, not true, or taken out of context, correct me. If you have ideas of how this book might be made better or if you have additional information or a personal experience that might be useful to me in my work, please write.

And if this book speaks to you in some special way, I'd like to know that, too. You can write me c/o The Crossing Press, P.O. Box 1048, Freedom, CA 95109.

Resources

Organizations

Alternative Bris Support Group
c/o Helen Bryce
P.O. Box 1305
Capitola, CA 95010-1305
Tel: 408-475-3313 (leave phone number, not just address)
Info and support.

Attorneys for the Rights of the Child
Attn: J. Steven Svoboda
2961 Ashby Avenue
Berkeley, CA 94705
Tel: 510-848-4437
E-mail: svoboda1@flash.net

Association for Pre- and Perinatal Psychology & Health
P.O. Box 994
Geyserville, CA 95441
Tel: 707-857-4041
E-mail: apppah@aol.com
Web: www.birth-psychology.com

Circumcision Resource Center (CRC)
Jewish Associates of CRC
P.O. Box 232
Boston, MA 02133
Tel/Fax: 617-523-0088
Ronald Goldman, Ph.D., Executive Director
E-mail: crc@ziplink.net
Web: www.circumcision.org

Doctors Opposing Circumcision (DOC)
2442 NW Market Street S-42
Seattle, WA 98107
Attn: George Denniston, M.D.
Web: weber.u.washington.edu/~gcd/DOC/
Primarily for doctors.

The Israeli Association Against Genital Mutilation/
Ha'amuta neged chituchim be'evrey hamin
P.O. Box 56178
Tel Aviv 61560, Israel
Tel: 972-3-639-4569 (Dr. Avshalom Zoossmann-Diskin)
E-mail: zoossmann@hotmail.com

Lightfoot Associates
4910 N. Calle Bosque
Tucson, AZ 85718
Tel: 520-529-2029
Fax: 520-529-9411
Attn: Hanny Lightfoot-Klein
E-mail: lobiond@primenet.com
Web: www.ibp.com/usa/lightfoot/
Female genital mutilation.

National Organization of Circumcision Information Resource Centers (NOCIRC)
P.O. Box 2512
San Anselmo, CA 94960
Tel: 415-488-9883
Fax: 415-488-9660
E-mail: nocirc@nbn.com
Web: www.nocirc.org

National Organization to Halt the Abuse and Routine Mutilation of Males (NOHARMM)
P.O. Box 460795
San Francisco, CA 94146
Tel: 415-826-9351
Fax: 415-642-3700
Web: www.noharmm.org

National Organization of Restoring Men (NORM)
c/o R. Wayne Griffiths
3205 Northwood Drive, Suite 209
Concord, CA 94520-4506
Tel: 510-827-4077
Fax: 510-827-4119
E-mail: waynerobb@aol.com
Web: www.norm.org
Foreskin restoration.

Nurses for the Rights of the Child
Attn: Betty Katz Sperlich, R.N., and Mary Conant, R.N.
369 Montezuma #354
Santa Fe, NM 87501
Tel: 505-989-7377

E-mail: wholebaby@nets.com
Web: www.cirp.org/nrc/
Source for *Handbook for R.N. Conscientious Objectors to Infant Circumcision* and *The Nurses of St. Vincent: Saying No to Circumcision* (video).

Further Reading

Circumcision: The Hidden Trauma—How An American Cultural Practice Affects Infants and Ultimately Us All, by Ronald Goldman, Ph.D. Toll-free orders: 888-445-5199.

Circumcision: The Rest of the Story. Mothering Magazine, P.O. Box 1690, Santa Fe, NM 87504. Tel: 505-984-8116.

The Joy of Uncircumcising! Restore Your Birthright and Maximize Sexual Pleasure, by Jim Bigelow, Ph.D., Hourglass Book Publishing, P.O. Box 171, Aptos, CA 95001. Available from UNCIRC, P.O. Box 52138, Pacific Grove, CA 93950. Tel: 408-375-4326

To Mutilate in the Name of Jehovah or Allah: Legitimization of Male and Female Circumcision, by Sami A. Aldeeb Abu-Sahlieh. From NOHARMM (see Organizations) or viewable at http://www.hollyfeld.org/~xastur/mutilate.html.

Questioning Circumcision: A Jewish Perspective, by Ronald Goldman. Toll-free orders: 888-445-5199.

Say No to Circumcision: 40 Compelling Reasons, by Thomas J. Ritter, M.D. and George C. Denniston, M.D. Hourglass Book Publishing, P.O. Box 171, Aptos, CA 95001.

Sexual Mutilations: A Human Tragedy, edited by George C. Denniston and Marilyn Fayre Milos, Plenum Press. Presentations at the Fourth International Symposium on Sexual Mutilations in Lausanne, Switzerland, August 9–11, 1996.

The Warrior's Journey Home: Healing Men's Addictions, Healing the Planet, by Jed Diamond. New Harbinger. Orders: 800-748-6273.

Video

Whose Body, Whose Rights? The premier video on the subject. Available from VideoFinders, 4401 Sunset Blvd., Los Angeles, CA 90027, order toll-free 800-343-4727.

World Wide Web

Circumcision Information and Resource Pages (CIRP)
Web: www.cirp.org/CIRP/

Circumcision, online peer-review medical journal
Robert S. van Howe, M.D., FAAP, editor.
Web: weber.u.washington.edu/~gcd/CIRCUMCISION/

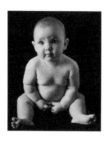

APPENDIX

NON-CIRCUMCISION
NOTIFICATION FORM

Copy the form on the following pages and present it to all the health care personnel who will come into contact with your baby after he is born—but do it well in advance of the birth. Most doctors, out of justifiable fear of lawsuits, will not circumcise a child if either parent objects. But you must make your objection very clear, especially if your partner favors circumcision or doesn't consider it very important one way or the other.

NON-CIRCUMCISION NOTIFICATION FORM

Attention: Maternal-Infant Care Staff, Physicians, Nurses, and other Personnel at:

Name of Facility:

_____

Address:

_____

(We, I, My spouse) plan(s) to use your maternal care facility for the purposes of childbirth, and hereby provide you with this notification that (our/my) male child **is not to be circumcised under any circumstances.**

To avoid potential error whereby this child could be circumcised, (we, I) hereby direct that the mother's chart be immediately marked upon admission, that the child's chart be marked immediately after birth, and that his nursery crib be very clearly marked:

Circumcision Forbidden
Do Not Retract or Manipulate Foreskin

(We, I) further direct that no attempt be made by anyone at this facility to stretch, retract, or otherwise forcibly manipulate our son's prepuce (foreskin).

(We, I) wish to accord this new child a full respect for his rights to physical integrity and eventual self-determination and to spare him any needless pain and potentially damaging iatrogenic interventions.

Important: (We, I) trust that these directions will be honored. Should any portion of this notice be disregarded, however, or should this child be circumcised based on any consent form not bearing dual consent from at least two of the following signatures [Mother/Father/Co-Parent/Legal Guardian], (we, I) reserve the right to take appropriate legal action(s).

This document becomes legally binding with at least one signature below.

Signature _____

Print Name _____

Relationship to child (check one): ___ Mother ___ Father
         ___ Co-Parent ___ Legal Guardian

Date: _____

Signature _____

Print Name _____

Relationship to child (check one): ___ Mother ___ Father
         ___ Co-Parent ___ Legal Guardian

Date: _____

Text provided by National Organization to Halt the Abuse and Routine Mutilation of Males: PO Box 460795, San Francisco, CA 94146. Tel: 415-826-9351, Fax: 415-646-3700

MALE HEALTH & GENITAL CARE

Previous Circumcision Rationale and Modern Alternatives

Urinary Tract Infection (UTI)

Prophylaxis: Breastfeeding[1]; rooming-in[2]; avoiding premature foreskin retraction reduces risk of exposing urinary opening to fetal bacteria.

Treatment: Antimicrobial therapy.[3]

Phimosis, Adhesions

Diagnosis inappropriate before completion of penile development (full preputial separation from glans may not occur until late adolescence.[4-7])

Treatment: Topical steroid cream at preputial orifice resolves phimosis[8-10]; lysis resolves adhesions.[11]

Paraphimosis

Prophylaxis: Teach adults to "leave the foreskin alone."[12]; Age-appropriate materials exist to teach children not to prematurely retract prepuce beyond what is comfortable.[13,14]

Treatment: Compress glans with fingers, slip foreskin forward.[15] Hyaluronidase also reduces swelling.[16]

Balanitis, Posthitis, or Balanoposthitis

Prophylaxis: Avoid exposure to soled diapers, bubble baths, soap on genitals/in clothing, chlorinated water; eat yogurt to replenish microbial flora after antibiotic therapy; drink water to reduce uric acid concentration.[17]

Treatment: Use of topical antimicrobials or effective herbal remedies.[18]

Risk Reduction for STDs, HIV/AIDS, and Genital Cancers (penis/cervix)

Prophylaxis: Encourage safer sex behaviors (avoid sex with infected partners, limit number of sexual partners if status is unknown, use condoms; practice good genital hygiene).[19, 20]; limit/avoid smoking.[21]

Improved Hygiene

Prophylaxis: No special hygienic intervention is warranted in children. In adults, smegma is a sexual emollient[22] and hygiene for both sexes is best accomplished with plain water (and soap, if tolerated).[12,17,23]

Zipper Entrapment

Prophylaxis: Instruct caution with zippers.   Treatment: Cut bottom of zipper, open upward.[24,25]

Aesthetics, Peer Conformity, Social Custom, Family Tradition or Religion

On ethical[26–28] and human rights grounds,[29–33] non-therapeutic circumcision is best decided by the person whose body it affects. Physicians are obliged to refrain from performing non-medically indicated circumcisions on persons who are unable to consent.[33,34] Religious circumcisions are done outside hospitals, one week or more after birth. Complications caused by unskilled operators are handled by the legal system.[34] Genital cutting of children by physicians acting as the agents of social custom compromises the physician's duty to protect the health and rights of those with no social power to protect themselves.[33]

Text provided by Doctors Opposing Circumcision, 2442 N.W. Market St., S-42, Seattle, WA 98107 USA

ENDNOTES

Circumcision, An Overview

1   Estimated by Robert van Howe, M.D., in his as yet unpublished cost/utility analysis, which takes into account both the cost of performing the circumcisions and the cost of treating complications.

2   Williams, N. and L. Kapila, "Complications of Circumcision," British Journal of Surgery, vol. 80, no 10, October 1993, pages 1231–1236: "Some authors have reported a complication rate as low as 0.06 percent, while at the other extreme rates of up to 55 percent have been quoted. This reflects differing and varying diagnostic criteria employed; a realistic figure is 2–10 percent."

3   On masthead of The Victims Speak, newsletter (no longer published) of The Victims Speak, from unpublished 1989 book manuscript by Marilyn Fayre Milos, R.N., Director, National Organization of Circumcision Information Resource Centers.

4   Fleiss, Paul M., M.D., "Where Is My Foreskin: The Case Against Circumcision," Mothering: The Magazine of Natural Family Living, No. 85, Winter 1997, pp. 36–45.

5   Letter received by The Victims Speak, dated 19 October 1988.

6   Taylor, J. R., A. P. Lockwood, and A .J. Taylor, Department of Pathology, Health Sciences Centre, University of Manitoba, Winnipeg, Manitoba, Canada, "The Prepuce: Specialized Mucosa of the Penis and Its Loss to Circumcision," British Journal of Urology, 1996, 77, 291–295.

7   Romberg, Rosemary, correspondence with the author, January 1990.

8   "Clinic-based Investigation of the Typology and Self-reporting of FGM in Egypt," November 1996, by the Egyptian Fertility Care Society, the Population Council, and Macro International. Summary

received by the author as e-mail from NOHARMM, October 14, 1997. The complete document may be scanned onto a home page on the World Wide Web.

9 From chart "Child-Victims of Genital Mutilation," by Ad Hoc Working Group of International Experts on Violations of Genital Mutilation, Copyright ©1995 by Ecumenics International USA.

10 Romberg, p. 3.

11 Bryk, Felix, *Sex and Circumcision: A Study of Phallic Worship and Mutilation in Men and Women*, Brandon House, North Hollywood, California, 1967, p. 80, cited by Romberg, p. 3.

12 Eltahawy, Mona, "Group Sues Muslim Leaders over Female Circumcision," Reuters News Service, July 8, 1995. The head of al-Azhar is Sheikh Gad el-Haq Ali Gad el-Haq.

13 An e-mail received by the author from Sami Aldeeb, Staff Advisor for Arab and Islamic Law, Swiss Institute of Comparative Law, on December 30, 1997, citing statements made to him by Dr. Seham Abdel-Salam, whose organization had spearheaded the legal drive to have female circumcision declared illegal by the Egyptian high court.

14 Daly, Mary, *Gyn Ecology: The Metaphysics of Radical Feminism*, "The Sacred Passage," Ch. 5, "African Genital Mutilation: The Unspeakable Atrocities," p. 165. Her reference: Henny Harald Hansen, "Clitoridectomy: Female Circumcision in Egypt," Folk, Vol. 14–15, 1972/73, p. 18.

15 Information on response to female circumcision in Britain, Italy, and France from a conversation (1989) between the author and Marilyn Fayre Milos, Director, National Organization of Circumcision Information Resource Centers, based on a telephone conversation between her and Fran Hosken, Women's International Network.

16 From interview on "New Paradigms" program hosted by Maureen Primerano, broadcast on KMUD, Garberville, California, December 26, 1996. Transcribed and supplied to the author by Tim Hammond of NOHARMM.

17 Toubia, Nahid, M.D., "FGM and the Responsibility of Reproductive Health Professionals," *International Journal of Gynecology & Obstetrics*, 46, 1994, pp. 127–135.

18 Adapted from a flyer from the National Organization Against the Routine Mutilation of Males (NOHARMM).

"Medical" Basis for Circumcision

1 Spratling, E. J., "Masturbation in the Adult," *Medical Record*, 1895; 45:442–3. Quoted by Frederick Hodges, "A Short History of the Institutionalization of Involuntary Sexual Mutilation in the United States," paper presented at the Fourth International Symposium on Sexual Mutilations, Lausanne, Switzerland, August 9–11, 1996.

2 Kellogg, John Harvey. *Plain Facts for Old and Young.* New edition, revised and enlarged. I.F. Segner & Co., Burlington, Iowa, 1888, pp. 294–295.

3 Resner, Paul, "Tissue Helps Skin's Healing Process," AP Science Writer, Associated Press, October 20, 1997.

4 Hodges, F. A., "Short History of the Institutionalization of Involuntary Sexual Mutilation in the United States," in G .C. Denniston and M. F. Milos, eds., *Sexual Mutilations: A Human Tragedy*, Plenum Press, New York, 1997, p. 35, cited by Paul A. Fleiss, M.D., "Where Is My Foreskin: The Case Against Circumcision," *Mothering*, No. 85, Winter 1997, p. 39.

5 King, Lowell R., M.D., "The Pros and Cons of Neonatal Circumcision" (unpublished), cited by Romberg, Rosemary, in *Circumcision: The Painful Dilemma*, Bergin & Garvey, South Hadley, MA, 1985, p. 274.

6 Ravich, A., "The Relationship of Circumcision to Cancer of the Prostate," *Journal of Urology*, Vol. 48, 1942, p. 298–299, cited by Romberg, Rosemary, in *Circumcision: The Painful Dilemma*, Bergin & Garvey, South Hadley, MA, 1985, p. 255.

7 Stagg, Del, P.D., "A Basis for Decision on Circumcision," from *Compulsory Hospitalization or Freedom of Choice in Childbirth?, Vol. III* (Transcripts of the 1978 NAPSAC Convention—Stewart & Stewart) Ch. 63, p. 833, cited by Romberg, Rosemary, in *Circumcision: The Painful Dilemma*, p. 257.

8 Winberg, Jan, M.D., Ingela Bollgren, M.D., Leif Gothefors, M.D., Maria Herthelius, M.D., and Kjell Tullus, M.D., "The Prepuce: A Mistake of Nature?" *The Lancet*, March 18, 1989.

9 Based on e-mail to the author from medical historian Frederick Hodges at Oxford University, discussing the paper by George C. Denniston, M.D., "Circumcision: An Iatrogenic Epidemic," presented at the Fourth International Symposium on Sexual Mutilations in Lausanne, Switzerland, August 9–11, 1996.

10 "UTI Studies Refuted," *NOCIRC Newsletter*, National Organization of Circumcision Information Resource Centers, Vol. 4, No. 1, Winter 1989–90, p. 2.

11 Marino, Leonard J., M.D., "An Emphatic Vote against Circumcision," letter to *Contemporary Pediatrics*, November 1989, pp. 11, 14.

12 Romberg, Rosemary, personal correspondence with author, January 1990.

13 Gellis, Sydney, M.D., *American Journal of Diseases of Childhood*, Vol. 132, December 1978, p. 1168, cited in Romberg, Rosemary, *Circumcision: The Painful Dilemma*, p. 247.

14 Fleiss, Paul, M.D., "Care of the Intact Penis," *NOCIRC Newsletter*, Vol. 4, No. 1, Winter 1989–90, p 2.

15 Marck, J., "Aspects of Male Circumcision in Sub-equatorial African Culture," *Health Transition Review 1997*; 7, Suppl, pp. 337–59.

16 Robert Van Howe, M.D., in e-mail to the author, September 29, 1997, citing the following six largest studies mentioned in the quote:

Chao, A., M. Bulterys, F. Musanganire, P. Habimana, P. Nawrocki, E. Taylor, A. Dushimimana, A. Saah, "Risk Factors Associated with Prevalent HIV-1 Infection among Pregnant Women in Rwanda," National University of Rwanda-Johns Hopkins University AIDS Research Team. *International Journal of Epidemiology*, 1994; 23: 371–80.

Barongo L.R., M.W. Borgdorff, F.F. Mosha, A. Nicoll, H. Grosskurth, K.P. Senkoro, J.N. Newell, J. Changalucha, A.H. Klokke, J.Z. Killewo, J.P. Velema, R.J. Hayes, D.T. Dunn, L.A.S. Muller, J.B. Rugemalila, "The Epidemiology of HIV-1 Infection in Urban Areas, Roadside Settlements and Rural Villages in Mwanza Region, Tanzania," *AIDS* 1992, 6:1521–8.

Grosskurth H., F. Mosha, J. Todd, K. Senkoro, J. Newell, A. Klokke, J. Changalucha, B. West, P. Mayaud, A. Gavyole, R. Gabone, D. Mabey,

R. Hayes, "A Community Trial of the Impact of Improved Sexually Transmitted Disease Treatment on the HIV Epidemic in Rural Tanzania: 2. Baseline Survey Results," *AIDS*, 1995, 9:927–34.

Van de Perre P., M. Carael, D. NzVanaramba, G. Zissis, J. Kayihigi, J.P. Butzler, "Risk Factors for HIV Seropositivity in Selected Urban-based Rwandese Adults," *AIDS*, 1987, 1:207–11.

Quigley M., K. Munguti, H. Grosskurth, J. Todd, F. Mosha, K. Senkoro, J. Newell, P Mayaud, F. ka-Gina, A. Klokke, D. Mabey, A. Gavyole, R. Hayes, "Sexual Behaviour Patterns and Other Risk Factors for HIV in Rural Tanzania: A Case-Control Study," *AIDS*, 1997, 11:237–48.

Urassa M., J. Todd, J.T. Boerma, R. Hayes, R. Isingo, "Male Circumcision and the Susceptibility to HIV Infection among Men in Tanzania," *AIDS*, 1997, 11:73–80.

For more on the 28 existing studies that together implicate circumcision more than intactness as predisposing toward HIV infection, see: Van Howe, R.S., "An Objective Assessment of Neonatal Circumcision," *American Academy of Pediatrics Task Force on Circumcision*, Rosemont, Illinois, June 8, 1997; or Van Howe, R.S., "Circumcision and HIV-Infections: Review of the Literature and Meta-analysis; Under Consideration.

17 Desantis, George, "Circumcision: Prime Cut," *QQ Magazine* (no longer published), March/April 1976, cited by John Erickson, Gulf Coast Infant Circumcision Information Center, May 1987 mailing.

18 "Circumcision Ban," *NOCIRC Newsletter*, Vol. 4, No. 1, Winter 1989–90, p. 2.

19 "Canadian Paediatric Society Upholds Anti-circumcision Stand," *NOCIRC Newsletter*, Vol. 4, No. 1, Winter 1989–90, p. 2.

20 Romberg, p. 248.

21 From a letter written by John P. Hansen, M.D., M.S.P.H., Medical Director, Group Health Cooperative, One South Park Street, Madison, Wisconsin 53715, dated March 23, 1994.

22 From a letter written by W. Knox Fitzpatrick, M.D., Vice President of Medical Affairs, Blue Cross Blue Shield of Utah, 2455 Parley's Way, P.O. Box 30270, Salt Lake City, UT 84130-0270, dated September 21, 1994.

23 From Dr. Snyder's presentation at the First International Symposium on Circumcision, March 1–3, 1989, Anaheim, California. The author was in attendance.

24 Fink, Aaron J., M.D., *Circumcision: A Parent's Decision for Life*, Kavanah Publishing, Los Altos, CA, 1988.

25 *Ibid.* p. 12.

26 Original citation lost. Referred to in "Circumcision's Comeback?", Family Report by Vicki Brower, *American Health*, September 1989, p. 126, in which Ms. Bower implies that the AAP "recommends" that parents take these factors into account, not that they simply observe that they do.

27 Letter reprinted in *NOCIRC Newsletter*, circa 1988.

28 "Washington State Saves Health-care Dollars," *NOCIRC Newsletter*, Vol. 4, No. 1, Winter 1989–90, p. 2.

29 Fink, p. 17.

30 *Ibid.*, p. 1.

31 Trager, James, "Media Distorts AAP Report," *Medical Tribune*, June 8, 1989, cited by *NOCIRC Newsletter*, Vol. 4., No. 1, Winter 1989–90, p. 1.

32 Collected by the National Organization of Circumcision Information Resource Centers.

33 Brower, Vicki, "Circumcision's Comeback?", Family Report, *American Health*, September 1989, p. 126.

34 "AAP Alters Position and Confuses Parents," *NOCIRC Newsletter*, Romberg, Rosemary, correspondence with the author, January 1990, Vol. 4, No. 1, Winter 1989–90, p. 1.

35 Kirkey, Sharon, "Circumcising Baby Boys 'Criminal Assault,' Ethicist Says Society Must Consider Ban," *The Ottawa Citizen*, Friday, October 17, 1997. Article at http://www.ottawacitizen.com/national/971017/1263272.html.

Religious Basis for Circumcision

1 Wrana, Phoebe, "Circumcision," *Historical Review*,p. 387, cited by Romberg, p. 88.

2   Anonymity requested.

3   From materials sent out by an Alternative Bris Support Group, 1989.

4   Wallerstein, Edward, "Circumcision and Anti-Semitism: An Update," *Humanistic Judaism* (undated photocopy).

5   Romberg, p. 10, re: tribal societies in Australia and New Guinea.

6   Bettelheim, Bruno, *Symbolic Wounds: Puberty Rites and the Envious Male*, Thames and Hudson, London, 1955. Out of print. (Available through inter-library loan.)

7   Maimonides, Moses, *The Guide for the Perplexed*, as quoted in "The Development of Circumcision in Judaism," *The Joy of Uncircumcising*, by Jim Bigelow, Ph.D., Hourglass Book Publishing, Aptos, CA.

8   Phone conversation with the author, mid-October 1988. Anonymity requested.

9   Briggs, Anne, *Circumcision: What Every Parent Should Know*, p. 172., 1985

10 Flyer received in the mail by the author in 1989 from a circumcisionist, as evidence that the preservationist movement was racist.

11 Rabbi Burt Jacobson (Jewish Renewal Movement), Kehilla Synagogue, Oakland/Berkeley, California. Interview with the author, June 1989.

12 Written statement received by The Victims Speak, undated, summer 1988.

13 Interview by author with Rabbi Burt Jacobson (Jewish Renewal Movement), Kehilla Synagogue, Oakland/Berkeley, California, June 1989.

14 Romberg, p. 55.

15 Karsenty, Nelly, "A Mother Questions Brit Milla," *Humanistic Judaism*, Summer 1988, p. 14.

16 "Jewish Feminists Prompt Protests at Wailing Wall" (with photo), *New York Times*, December 2, 1988, p. A10, quoting Rabbi Meir Yehuda Getz (Orthodox).

17 From an addendum in *Questioning Circumcision: A Jewish Perspective*, by Ronald Goldman, Ph.D., based on a May 5, 1997 news item that appeared on the SNS News Service (Israel); Vanguard, Boston, 1997.

Healing Our Culture, Healing Ourselves

1 From interview in NOHARMM newsletter, July 1997.

2 Letter received by the National Organization of Circumcision Information Resource Centers.

3 Undated and uncredited newspaper clipping received in the mail by the author on February 26, 1990, from a medical advice column by "Dr. Lamb," © 1985, News American Syndicate.

4 Abbott, Franklin, "What To Do When Shit Happens: Reaction and Responsibility," Health and Healing section, *Southern Voice*, 1989 (undated photocopy).

5 Nancy Mulnix, RN, MA, "Managed Pain," *Informant*, newsletter of NOCIRC of Michigan, P.O. Box 333, Birmingham, MI 48012, Tel: 248-642-5703, p. 1.

6 Nancy Mulnix, R.N., "Managed Pain: Will Michigan Hear the Screams of Babies?", *The Informant*, newsletter of NOCIRC of Michigan, September 1997, p. 1.

7 "Circumcised Men Want It All Back," Sex Matters advice column by Louanne Cole Weston, Ph.D., *San Francisco Examiner*, Wednesday, October 15, 1997, p. C-7. E-mail received by author from NOHARMM on October 16, 1997. Weston is a board-certified sex therapist and licensed marriage and relationship counselor with offices in San Francisco and Sacramento. Send questions to: Sex Matters, Style, *San Francisco Examiner*, P.O. Box 7260, San Francisco, CA 94120, or e-mail to: lcole@ix.netcom.com.

8 In a letter to NOHARMM, March 14, 1993.

9 Marcello, P. C., "Foreskin Restoration: What Is It?", accompanying article to "Circumcision: the Unkindest Cut?", *Sex Life*, Vol. 2, Zygote, Inc., 530 Showers Drive #7-315, Mountain View, CA 94040, e-mail: zygote@fugue.com.

10 "Working Together for Children's Rights," May 1989, International Save the Children Alliance, 147 rue de Lausanne, CH-1202 Geneva, Switzerland, p. 2, "Basic Principles."

11 "High Court Awards Scarred Child £10,000," *NOCIRC Newsletter*, Vol. 4, No. 1, Winter 1989–90.

12 Letter received January 1989 by the National Organization of Circumcision Information Resource Centers.

13 "Statement of Principles and Purpose," The Victims Speak, undated, circa 1988.

14 From the introductory talk at which Marilyn Milos was presented the Maurine Ricke Award for Clinical Excellence in Perinatal Nursing, California Nurses' Association, Region 9, April 1988.

15 Speaking on *Talk of the Nation*, National Public Radio, November 9, 1993.

16 Badawi, Mohammed, M.D., M.P.H., First International Symposium on Circumcision, March 1–3, 1989, Anaheim, California. The author was in attendance.

17 Cited, unreferenced, in an issue of *The Vegan* magazine (UK).

Appendix

1 Piscane, A. et al., "Breastfeeding and Urinary Tract Infection," *Journal of Pediatrics*, 1992;120:87–9.

2 Winberg, J. et al., "The Prepuce: A Mistake of Nature?", *Lancet*, 1989; 1:598–9.

3 McCracken, G., "Options in Antimicrobial Management of UTI in Infants and Children," *Pediatric Infectious Disease Journal*, 1989; 8:8552–5.

4 Gairdner, D. "Fate of the foreskin," *British Medical Journal*, 1949;2:1433–7.

5 Øster, J., "Further Fate of the Foreskin," *Archives of Disease in Childhood*, 1968;43:200–3.

6 Catzel, P., "The Normal Foreskin in the Young Child," *SA Mediese Tydskrif*, 1982;62:751.

7 Hayabe, H., "Analysis of Shape and Retractability of the Prepuce in 603 Japanese Boys," *Journal Urology*, 1996;156:1813–5.

8 Wright, J.E., "The Treatment of Childhood Phimosis with Topical Steroid," *Australian-New Zealand Journal of Surgery*, 1994;64:327–8.

9   Jorgenson, E.T., "The Treatment of Phimosis in Boys with a Potent Topical Steroid (Clobetasol Propionate 0,05%) Cream," *Acta Dermato-Venereologica*, 1993;73:55–6.

10 Golubovic, A. et al., "The Conservative Treatment of Phimosis in Boys," *British Journal of Urology*, 1995;78:786–8.

11 MacKinlay, G.A., "Save the Prepuce: Painless Separation of Preputial Adhesions in the Outpatient Clinic," *British Medical Journal*, 1988; 297:590–1.

12 AAP, *Newborns: Care of the Uncircumcised Penis*. (brochure) American Academy of Pediatrics, 1994.

13 Jensen, J., *"Good News for Boys: A Newspaper for Intact Boys,"* J.C. Jensen, M.S.W., PO Box 584, Tacoma, WA 98401-0584.

14 Noble, E., *The Joy of Being a Boy!*, New Life Images, 448 Pleasant Lake Ave., Harwich, MA 02645; 1994.

15 Illingworth, R., *The Normal Child: Some Problems of the Early Years and Their Treatment*, Churchill Livingston, 1983: 101.

16 DeVries, C., "Reduction of Paraphimosis with Hyaluronidase," *Urology*, 1996;48:464–5.

17 NOCIRC. *Answers to your questions about your young son's intact penis*. (brochure) National Organization of Circumcision Information Resource Centers, PO Box 2512, San Anselmo, CA 94970; 1996.

18 Green, J., "Penis-Foreskin Inflammation," in *The Male Herbal: Health Care for Men and Boys*, The Crossing Press, Freedom, CA 1991; 116–25.

19 Poland, R., "The Question of Routine Neonatal Circumcision," *New England Journal of Medicine*, 1990;322:1312–14.

20 Frisch, M., et al., "Falling Incidence of Penile Cancer in an Uncircumcised Population," *British Medical Journal*, 1995;311:1471.

21 Harish, K., "The Role of Tobacco in Penile Carcinoma," *British Journal of Urology*, 1995;75:385–7.

22 Wright, J., "How Smegma Serves the Penis," *Sexology*, 170;37:50–53.

23 Kreuger, H., "Effects of Hygiene among the Uncircumcised," *Journal Family Practice*, 1986;22:353–5.

24 Flowerdew, R. et al., "Management of Penile Zipper Injury," *Journal of Urology*, 1977;117:671.

25 Chaflin, L., "Win One from the Zipper," *Emergency Medicine*, 1989;21:96.

26 AAP Committee on Bioethics, "Informed Consent: Parental Permission and Assent in Pediatric Practice," *Pediatrics*, 1995;95:314–7.

"A patient's reluctance or refusal to assent should carry considerable weight when the proposed intervention is not essential to his or her welfare and/or can be deferred without substantial risk. Providers have legal and ethical duties to child patients to render medical care based on what the patient needs, not what someone else expresses."

27 Denniston, G., "Circumcision and the Code of Ethics," *Humane Health Care International*, April, 1996:12.

"Circumcision Violates All Seven Principles of Medical Ethics (AMA 1992)."

28 Thompson, R., "Routine Circumcision in the Newborn: An Opposing View," *Journal Family Practice*, 1990; 31:189–96.

29 LeBourdais, E., "Circumcision No Longer a "Routine" Surgical Procedure," *Canadian Medical Assoc. Journal*, 1995;11:1873–6.

30 Phillips, I., "Advocacy: Rhetoric or Practice," *Nursing BC*, 1994;37–8.

"Circumcision is an issue of self-determination and autonomy. Circumcisions done for the personal preference or religion of the parent(s) are not in the best interests of the infant."

31 Milso, M., and D. Macris, "Circumcision: Medical or Human Rights Issue?", *Journal Nurse-Midwifery*, 1992; 37:suppl. 87S-96S.

32 Katz-Sperlich, B., and M. Conant, R.N., "Conscientious Objectors to Infant Circumcision: A model for Nurse Empowerment," *Revolution-Journal of Nurse Empowerment*, Spring 1996;86–9.

33 Toubia, N., "FGM and Responsibility of Reproductive Health Professionals," *International Journal Obstetrics & Gynecology*, 1994;46: 127–35.

"The unnecessary removal of a functioning body organ in the name of tradition, custom, or any other non-disease related cause should never be acceptable to the health profession. All childhood circum-

cisions are violations of human rights and a breach of the fundamental code of medical ethics. In many societies, health professionals
have successfully opposed ritual and other customary bodily mutilations. It is the moral duty of educated professionals to protect the
health and rights of those with little or no social power to protect
themselves."

34 Wallerstein, E., "Circumcision: Ritual Surgery or Surgical Ritual?",
Medicine and Law, 1983;2:85–97

"If a suit is brought (against a religious circumciser), this becomes a
secular matter for the courts to decide. The medical profession in the
U.S. has not put its own house in order. Newborn non-religious circumcision has no place in a rational society and should cease."

RELATED BOOKS FROM THE CROSSING PRESS

The Male Herbal: Health Care for Men & Boys
By James Green

"A wealth of information on topics most herbal books don't touch—men's sexual and emotional health—recommended for alternative health care collections."

—*Library Journal*

$14.95 • Paper • 0-89594-458-8

Natural Healing for Babies & Children
By Aviva Jill Romm

This is an indispensable volume for parents seeking safe and effective ways to promote and maintain their child's health using herbal and other natural remedies.

$16.95 • Paper • 0-89594-786-2

The Natural Pregnancy Book:
Herbs, Nutrition, and Other Holistic Choices
By Aviva Jill Romm

Aviva Jill Romm describes natural techniques, herbal remedies, and nutritional aids to support a healthy pregnancy for the woman who wants to take a proactive role in her prenatal care.

$19.95 • Paper • 0-89594-819-2

Pocket Guide to Midwifery Care
By Aviva Jill Romm

If you are pregnant, plan to be pregnant, or are curious about alternatives to medical childbirth, this Pocket Guide will provide you with complete information about midwifery care.

$6.95 • Paper • 0-89594-855-9

To receive a current catalog from The Crossing Press,
please call toll-free, 800-777-1048.
Visit our Website on the Internet at: www.crossingpress.com